Study Guide to Accompany
Radiologic Physics

Study Guide to Accompany
Radiologic Physics

Mosby's Radiographic Instructional Series

with illustrations

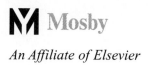 Mosby

An Affiliate of Elsevier

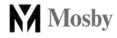

An Affiliate of Elsevier

Editor: Jeanne Rowland
Developmental Editor: Carole Glauser
Director, Media Production: Guy Jacobs
Project Manager: Gayle May Morris
Production Editor: Pam Martin
Manufacturing Manager: Patricia Stinecipher

Printed in the United States of America
Editorial services provided by Tom Lochhaas
Composition by Black Dot

Mosby
11830 Westline Industrial Drive
St. Louis, MO 63146

ISBN-13: 978-0-8151-5405-1
ISBN-10: 0-8151-5405-4

07 08 / 9 8 7 6 5 4

Introduction

Radiologic Physics Study Guide is designed to accompany the Radiologic Physics multimedia program in *Mosby's Radiographic Instructional Series.* This study guide can be used with either the slide/audiotape or the CD-ROM version of the program. The multimedia portion of this instructional program, along with the study guide, will provide a solid foundation in the principles of physics in general and in specific applications to x-rays and x-ray equipment. The program can be used for both instruction and review.

The eight modules in this study guide correspond to the eight modules of the multimedia program. Usually you will find it more effective to experience the multimedia program first and then read and work through the accompanying module in the study guide. The different parts of each module in the study guide allow you to review and apply what you learn from the multimedia module as much or as little as you find helpful. Answers to the various exercises appear at the end of each module in the study guide.

Self-Assessment Pretest is a group of 10 multiple-choice questions designed to help you determine how much of the module's material you have already mastered from the multimedia program before beginning to review this material in the study guide. If you incorrectly answered some questions, pay more attention to those subjects as you proceed through the other parts of the study guide.

Key Terms is a brief glossary section that defines important terms introduced in the multimedia module. It is important to gain a clear understanding of these terms and the concepts they represent before proceeding. Take a moment to read quickly through these definitions, and when you encounter items with which you are not yet comfortable, give special attention to their meaning. These terms will continue to be used in following parts, helping you become more familiar with them and their importance in radiography.

Topical Outline presents in a brief format the primary information and knowledge covered by the multimedia module. As when reading the key terms definitions, pay particular attention to areas you are not confident you understand.

Review gives you a chance to interact with the material that has been briefly introduced through the Key Terms and Topical Outline sections. You are encouraged to write in the terms and phrases indicated by the blank lines in these descriptive and explanatory statements. Do not view this as a test. What is important in this exercise is that you are becoming more familiar with the terminology and concepts related to the module's content. Some artwork is included in this section, usually a variation of illustrations used in the multimedia program, to enhance the learning and retention of important concepts or processes.

Learning Quiz is unique among the various parts in that it is not intended to be used by those who have worked through the CD-ROM version of the multimedia program in what is called the "student mode"—a student at the computer individually working through the learning program. In other words, you will want to complete this section if you viewed the slide/audio version or the CD-ROM program in "instructor" mode, without experiencing the program individually at the computer. If you have already worked through the full interactive program at the computer, you can, if you choose, skip over this section, which includes exercises you will already have experienced in the computer tutorial. On the other hand, repeating these exercises in the study guide format may be valuable as additional review. These exercises are designed to help you increase your mastery of the material by answering questions that require knowledge and understanding of key information that has been presented so far.

Applications addresses the module's concepts and information at a higher level by asking questions that require you to apply what you have learned in different situations or examples. This necessitates a fuller understanding of the material—how the principles of physics apply to the specific topic. These questions are in some ways the most "difficult" in the module because they involve more than just defining terms or repeating information. Take your time with these. If you have difficulty, return to the Key Terms and Outline to review. If you do well in answering these questions, you probably have a good grasp of the material in this module.

Posttest is the final section in each module in the study guide. It consists of an average of 20 multiple-choice questions designed to assess your understanding and retention of the information in the module after having worked through the preceding study guide sections. The answers to this section, unlike other sections, are not included in this study guide but are printed in the instructor's manual for the program—this is to allow your course instructor to use the posttest for more formal evaluation if desired.

This study guide is intended to make your learning experience more satisfying, while at the same time helping you learn, master, and remember what may be new or difficult material. The authors hope you find it an enjoyable experience.

Contents

General Principles

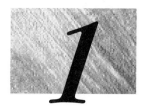

Self-Assessment Pretest

Use this pretest to assess your knowledge of the material in this module before you begin to work through the following exercises. Circle the best answer for each of the following questions. The answers are at the end of this module.

1. Which of the following is a fundamental unit of measurement?
   a. Length
   b. Volume
   c. Power
   d. Velocity

2. What two units of measurement are needed to determine momentum?
   a. Acceleration and time
   b. Speed and length
   c. Mass and velocity
   d. Distance and time

3. Two objects of equal mass but unequal size will have equal:
   a. Specific gravity
   b. Volume
   c. Density
   d. Weight

4. An object at rest is said to have:
   a. Friction
   b. Gravity
   c. Inertia
   d. Momentum

5. Mass times velocity is the mathematical calculation for:
   a. Acceleration
   b. Force
   c. Inertia
   d. Momentum

6. An object moving through the air can be slowed down by all of the following factors except:
   a. Mass
   b. Gravity
   c. Friction
   d. Impact

7. Force is applied to an object to increase or decrease its:
   a. Mass
   b. Acceleration
   c. Inertia
   d. Volume

8. Gravity is considered to be:
   a. Work
   b. Acceleration
   c. Power
   d. Inertia

9. The SI unit for work is:
   a. Joule
   b. Newton
   c. Work
   d. Watt

10. What type of energy does a boulder sitting on a mountain have?
    a. Mechanical
    b. Kinetic
    c. Potential
    d. Nuclear

Key Terms

Before continuing, be sure you can define the following key terms.

Absolute zero: the temperature point at which molecules are not moving at all; there is no kinetic energy of motion (heat).

Acceleration: a rate of change in velocity, measured in meters per second squared (m/sec^2). A positive acceleration results in increasing velocity, and a negative acceleration results in decreasing velocity.

Atom: the basic building block of matter that is made up of smaller particles called protons, neutrons, and electrons.

CGS system: a system of measurement that uses centimeters (cm), grams (g), and seconds.

Conduction: the direct transfer of heat from one object to another.

Convection: the process of heat transfer by a moving fluid or gas.

Density: the amount of mass in a certain amount of space or volume.

Derived unit: a unit are units of measurement that combines two or more fundamental units, such as volume, density, velocity, and specific gravity.

Energy: the ability to do work or make something happen. It can take the form of mechanical energy, heat, light, or electrical energy and is measured in the SI unit called the joule (J).

Force: the energy required to make an object move or to stop it from moving. Force (F) equals mass times acceleration.

Friction: the resistance caused by one object moving against or through another.

Fundamental unit: a unit that measures a quality by itself, without using any other fundamental unit, such as measure length, mass, time, and temperature; also called base unit or base quantity.

Gravity: the force of attraction between two objects with mass.

Inertia: the property of an object with mass to resist a change in its state of motion. Objects at rest will continue to stay at rest, and objects in motion will continue to move at the same velocity and direction.

Joule: the SI unit for work and energy; abbreviated as J.

Kelvin: the SI unit for temperature. The kelvin (K) scale begins at absolute zero.

Kinetic energy: the energy of an object in motion; abbreviated as KE.

Law of conservation of energy: The principle that energy is neither created nor destroyed but is only changed from one form to another.

Law of conservation of momentum: The principle that the momentum of an object in motion is not lost unless an outside force, such as friction or gravity, acts upon it.

Mass: abbreviated as the letter m and measured in kilograms (kg); dependent on the amount of matter in an object. Mass is similar to weight, but weight changes with the amount of gravity, while mass stays the same.

Matter: anything that exists in physical form; a solid, liquid, or gas.

MKS system: a system of measurement that uses meters (m), kg, and seconds.

Molecule: the smallest unit of a substance that retains the identity of that substance.

Momentum: abbreviated as the letter p; the product of mass (m) times velocity (v).

Newton: the SI unit for the amount of force (F) required to accelerate 1 kg at the rate of 1 m/sec^2; abbreviated as N.

Newton's second law of motion: The principle that the acceleration of an object is directly proportional to the amount of force applied.

Potential energy: stored energy by virtue of position; abbreviated as PE.

Power: the rate at which work is done, defined as work divided by time.

Radiation: a form of heat transfer from a warm object to the environment.

Rest energy: the energy all matter possesses because of its mass. All mass can be converted into energy through the formula $E = mc^2$, the mass of an object times the square of the speed of light.

SI unit: the internationally agreed-upon system of measurement. The system uses metric units as well as other agreed-upon scientific units, and measures such things as electric current, force, and energy.

Specific gravity: a comparison of the density of an object to the density of water. Water has a specific gravity of 1. Objects denser than water have a specific gravity higher than 1, and objects less dense than water have a specific gravity lower than 1.

Unit: a standard of measurement.

Velocity: the speed at which an object is moving. Velocity (v) is measured by determining the distance an object travels in a specific period of time. In the SI system velocity is measured in m/sec.

Volume: a measurement of space. It is a derived unit that requires combining two or more fundamental units.

Watt: the SI unit for power, abbreviated as W.

Weight: the force of gravity acting upon mass. As gravity changes, the mass of an object stays the same, but the weight of the object changes.

Work: the application of force to an object; the product of force times the distance the object is moved.

Topical Outline

The following material is covered in this module.

I. Standardized units of measurement are used in the sciences to determine and consistently express measurements of quantities and properties in physics.
    A. Fundamental units measure a quantity by themselves.
        1. Length is a fundamental unit expressed in meters.
        2. Mass is a fundamental unit expressed in kilograms.
        3. Time is a fundamental unit expressed in seconds.
        4. Temperature is a fundamental unit expressed in degrees K.
    B. Derived units combine two or more fundamental units.
        1. Volume is a derived unit that measures space.
        2. Density is a derived unit that measures the amount of mass in a certain amount of space.
        3. Velocity is a derived unit that measures the speed at which an object is moving.
        4. Specific gravity is a derived unit that measures the density of a substance compared to the density of water.
    C. The standard system of measurement agreed upon by scientists is called the SI system. It uses the metric system to measure distance and volume, seconds to measure time, watts (W) to measure power, joules to measure work, and degrees K to measure temperature.
II. The basic building block of all matter is the atom. The fundamental property of all matter, whether it is a gas, liquid, or solid, is that it has mass. Mass is the amount of matter in an object.
    A. Inertia is the property of an object with mass to resist a change in its state of motion.
    B. Momentum is the product of the mass times the velocity of the object.
        1. The law of conservation of momentum states that the momentum of an object in motion is not lost unless an outside force acts upon it.
III. Force equals mass times acceleration. Because of inertia, force is needed to make an object move and to stop an object that is already moving. Force can be imparted from one object to another.
    A. Mechanical force is used to overcome inertia by pushing or pulling an object.
        1. Acceleration is a change in velocity caused by the amount of force applied.
        2. Gravity is a force or acceleration that pulls all objects toward the earth at the same rate, 9.8 m/sec^2.
    B. Work is the term that physicists use for the application of force that moves an object. It is equal to force times the distance an object is moved.
        1. The joule is the derived unit of measurement for work.
    C. Power is the rate at which work is done. Mathematically, power is work divided by time.
        1. The watt is the unit of measurement for power.
IV. Energy is defined as the ability to do work.
    A. Potential energy is stored energy.
    B. Kinetic energy is the energy of an object in motion.
    C. The law of conservation of energy states that energy is neither created nor destroyed but is only changed from one form to another.

Review

1. Derived units are used in measurements that involve two or more fundamental units. For example, velocity is a derived unit that measures both distance (or length) and _time_.

Volume is a derived unit that is determined from three measurements of space: length, width, and height. The derived unit for _density_ requires measurements of both mass and volume.

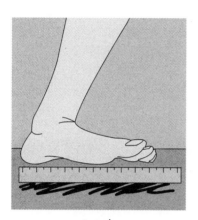

Length

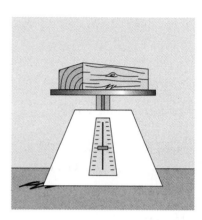

Mass

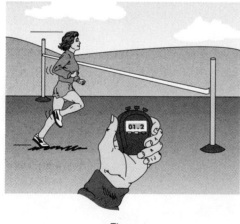

Time

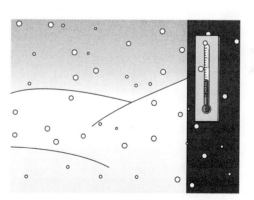

Temperature

Fundamental units

2. Velocity is the speed at which an object is moving. It is a __derived__ unit since it involves the measurement of how far an object moves in a period of time.

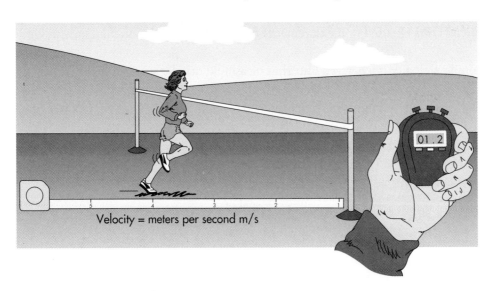

Velocity = meters per second m/s

3. The derived unit __Density__ is measured by the amount of mass in a certain amount of space or volume. When the density of a substance is compared to the density of water the result is a derived unit called __specific gravity__

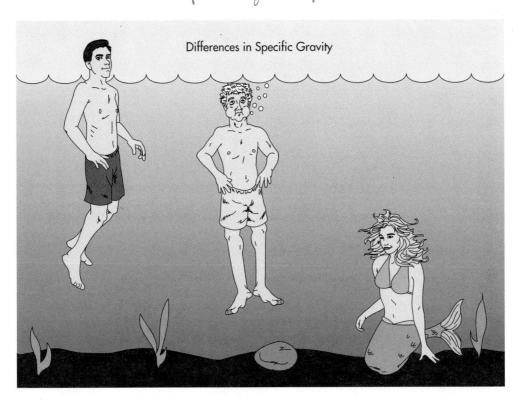

Differences in Specific Gravity

4. Of the two systems of measurement most commonly used around the world, the

   metric system is used by most scientists. In this system a kilometer (km) is 1000

   meter, a meter is 100 _centimeter_, and a centimeter is 10 _millimeter_.

5. In 1960 scientists agreed upon an international system of units called the

   SI units . This system measures mass in _kilograms_, time in _seconds_,

   temperature in _degrees K_, and electric current in _amperes_ .

6. Rocks, water, and baseballs are all composed of _matter_ .

7. Heat, light, electricity, and motors all are capable of making something happen. This ability to

   do work is the definition of _energy_ .

8. All substances, whether they are solid, liquid, or gas, are made up of atoms. Atoms are the

   basic building blocks of _matter_ . Atoms are composed of smaller particles called

   electrons, _protons_ , and _neutrons_ .

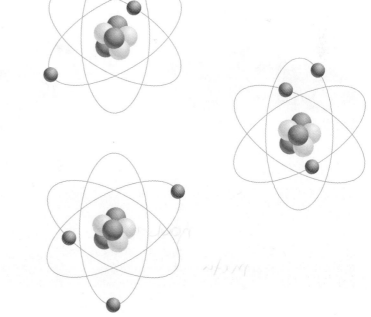

The Basic Building Blocks of Matter

9. A heavy rock has a large amount of __mass__ compacted into a small area. Air has a small amount of mass distributed in a __large__ area. The measurement for mass is __kilograms.__

10. Weight is often confused with mass, but weight is the force of __gravity__ acting upon mass.

11. The property of an object to resist change in its state of motion is __inertia__ and was described by Newton's first law of motion.

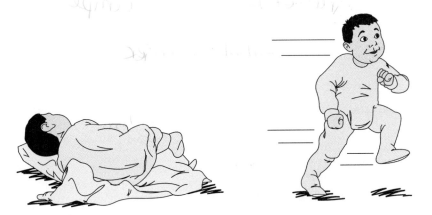

12. If a car were on a level surface it would theoretically continue rolling forever if it were not slowed down by __friction__. If brakes are applied to the wheels of the car, it can be said that __force__ is being used to overcome the car's __inertia__.

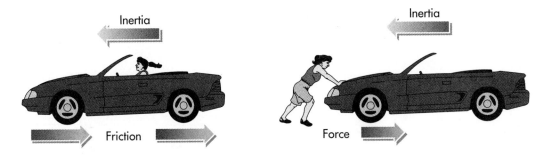

13. Both an object at rest and an object in motion have inertia. The object in motion has an additional characteristic called _momentum_, which is the result of mass times the _velocity_ at which the object is moving.

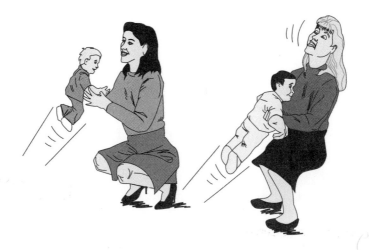

14. Imagine that a car with 1000 kg of mass is moving at 5 m/sec, and a second object of equal mass is moving at 10 m/sec. The faster-moving object will have twice as much _momentum_ as the first object.

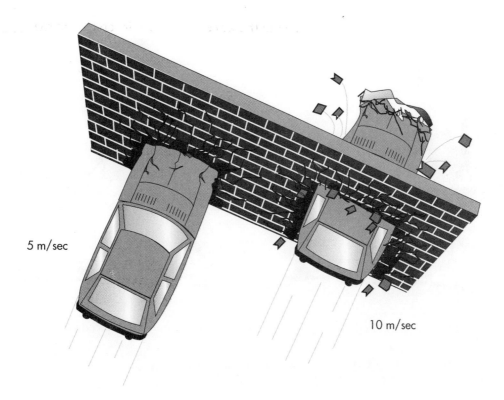

5 m/sec

10 m/sec

$$p = mv$$

15. The law of conservation of momentum states that the momentum resulting from an object in motion cannot be lost unless an outside _force_ acts upon it. Because of _inertia_, force is needed to start an object moving from a position at rest. Because of _momentum_, force is needed to stop an object that is already moving.

16. There are many kinds of force. The force of attraction between two objects with mass is _gravity_. The use of muscles provides _mechanical force_.

17. Newton's second law of motion states that _acceleration_ of a body by a force is directly proportional to the amount of force applied. Increasing velocity is _positive acceleration_, while decreasing velocity is _negative acceleration_.

18. By applying Newton's second law of motion you can determine the amount of acceleration. If you double the amount of _force_ pushing an object, the object will accelerate twice as fast. The mathematical formula for force is: force equals _mass_ times _acceleration_.

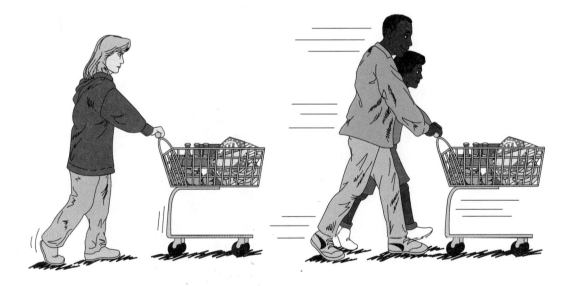

19. The SI unit for force is called the _newton_. This unit is the amount of force needed to accelerate 1 kg at the rate of one _meter_ per second per second.

20. _gravity_ pulls all objects to the earth with the same acceleration, 9.8 m/sec^2.

21. Physicists call the application of force to an object _work_. It is equal to the force times the _distance_ an object is moved. The SI unit for work is the _joule_.

22. The amount of work to move an object a certain distance is the same regardless of who or what does it. If one object is moved twice as fast as another object, the work is the same but the _power_ is different. Mathematically, this is equal to work divided by _time_. The SI unit for this is the _watt_.

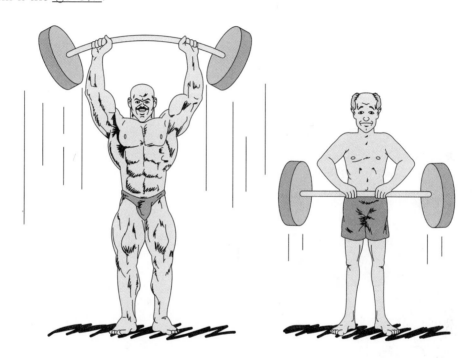

23. In physics the ability to do work is defined as _energy_. Mechanical work is the process of applying force to an object. Mechanical _energy_ is what enables movement to happen and it comes in two forms. _Kenetic_ energy is found in an object in motion, while _potential_ energy is stored energy.

24. The law of conservation of energy states that _energy_ cannot be created or destroyed but can only be changed from one form to another. Because of this the mechanical energy of muscles lifting an object is turned into _potential_ energy for the object.

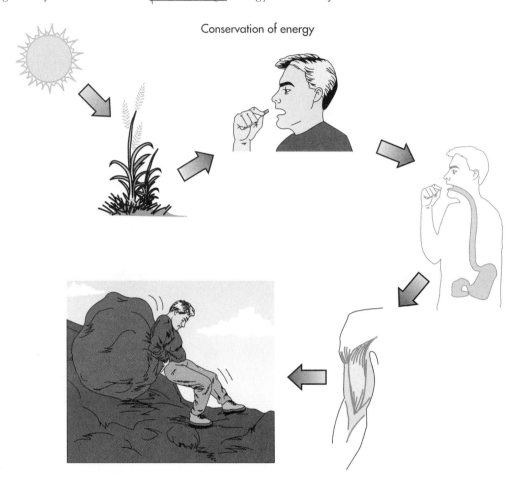

Conservation of energy

Learning Quiz

The following material is similar to the interactive exercises found in the CD-ROM version of this module operated in the "student mode." These questions will allow you to review the concepts presented in this module and will help you to gain a more complete understanding of the material.

1. Working with units of measurement often involves simple math to convert the units. This module uses a number of mathematical equations in its discussion of physics. Here is a quick question to warm up your mathematical brain cells. If there are 4 quarts (qt) in a gallon (gal), and there are 2 pints (pt) in a qt, how many pt are in 2 gal?

2. Let's get some more practice with math, using the example of velocity. The equation for velocity is $v = d/t$, or distance divided by time. Using this formula we can determine that a runner going 10 m in 2 seconds has a velocity of 5 m/sec. Keeping this in mind, if the velocity is 6 m/sec, how long will it take to run 42 m?

3. Think about matter for a moment. If you took a bottle of milk and poured all the milk out of it, would there be any matter left in the bottle?

4. A radiography student stands on an accurate hospital scale, his stomach growling with hunger. He is holding a pot containing 2 cups of water and a bag of uncooked rice. The scale says that he, along with what he is holding, weighs 160 pounds (lb).

Now he runs to a Bunsen burner in the chemistry lab, pours the rice into the water, boils it for 20 minutes, and eats every last grain of rice, which has absorbed the water in the pan. He then carries the empty pan back to the scale and stands on it.

Can you work this problem in your head? The water weighed 1.5 lb. The dry rice weighed 2 lb before it was cooked. The pan weighs 4 lb. (Assume that all the water was absorbed by the rice and none evaporated.)

What does the scale now say?
a. 158
b. 158.5
c. 160
d. 163.5

5. Here's a question on momentum. Imagine a pool table with three balls, one white and two red. If the white ball weighs 1 kg and is moving at 6 m/sec before it strikes the two red balls, it has a certain momentum. It imparts all that momentum to the two red balls, which weigh 1 and 2 kg each. If the 1-kg red ball moves away at 2 m/sec, what is the velocity of the 2-kg red ball?

6. This is a problem involving the calculation of work. How much work must you do to carry your textbooks up two flights of stairs? Let's say you have three books, each with a mass of 2 kg. Each flight of stairs has 11 steps. Each step is 20 cm high. Gravity exerts a force downward of 9.8 m/sec^2. Calculate the work needed to carry up the books.

7. Here's an interesting question. If a boulder fell off a cliff it would lose all its potential energy when it lost its height, and it would lose all its kinetic energy when it hit the ground and stopped moving. If energy is always conserved and can never be created or destroyed, where did the energy go?

Applications

1. If a man can run 1 km in 5 minutes, what is his velocity?

2. Imagine a man driving down an abandoned highway. The car he is driving has a mass of 900 kg. The man has a mass of 100 kg. As he travels down the highway at 10 m/sec he suddenly realizes that he is no longer on earth, but on a world with half the earth's gravity. At the moment of his realization he crashes into a brick wall. With how much momentum did the car strike the brick wall, in kg-m/sec?

3. On the last day of building Pharaoh's pyramid the chief engineer needed to calculate how much force would be needed to lift the 1000-kg cap stone. Determine how many newtons of force are required to raise the cap stone.

4. If the same chief engineer of Pharaoh's pyramid must raise the 1000-kg cap stone 300 m to the top of the pyramid, how much work is required?

5. Joe in the shipping department is able to lift a 10-kg box 10 m in 10 seconds on Monday. On Wednesday he is able to lift the same box 10 m in 5 seconds. What is the power that Joe uses on Monday and Wednesday?

6. While standing in an alley Joe looks up to see two large objects speeding toward him. Unable to get out of the way, he decides to jump in front of the object with the least momentum. Object A has a mass of 10 kg and is moving at 5 m/sec. Object B has a mass of 25 kg and is moving at 2 m/sec. Which object has the least momentum?

Posttest

Circle the best answer for each of the following questions. Your instructor has the correct answers.

1. Which of the following is *not* a fundamental unit of measurement?
   a. Length
   b. Mass
   c. Density
   d. Time

2. What two fundamental units of measurement are needed to determine velocity?
   a. Acceleration and time
   b. Speed and length
   c. Distance and time
   d. Distance and momentum

3. The density of a substance compared to the density of water is a measurement of:
   a. Specific gravity
   b. Volume
   c. Mass
   d. Space

4. What is the internationally agreed-upon system for measurement used by scientists?
   a. Metric units
   b. SI units
   c. MKS units
   d. CGS units

5. Which of the following is *not* true of matter? All matter has:
   a. Inertia
   b. Rest energy
   c. Mass
   d. Kinetic energy

6. The smallest unit of a substance that still has an identity of that substance is:
   a. An atom
   b. A molecule
   c. An element
   d. A proton

7. Two objects of equal mass have equal:
   a. Size
   b. Volume
   c. Density
   d. Weight

8. What is the property of an object that allows it to resist a change in its state of motion?
   a. Friction
   b. Gravity
   c. Inertia
   d. Mass

9. Momentum is calculated as a product of:
   a. Mass and acceleration
   b. Distance and time
   c. Mass and inertia
   d. Mass and velocity

10. Which of the following will *not* result in a loss of momentum in a moving object?
    a. Mass
    b. Gravity
    c. Friction
    d. Impact

11. Which of the following is *not* true of force?
    a. Force has mass.
    b. Force is needed to overcome inertia.
    c. Force is needed to stop momentum.
    d. Force can be imparted to another object.

12. Acceleration of a body is directly proportional to the amount of:
    a. Density
    b. Force applied
    c. Momentum
    d. Velocity

13. Gravity pulls objects toward the earth at a:
    a. Rate of 5.5 m/sec
    b. Rate of 9.8 m/sec^2
    c. Constant rate
    d. Rate of mass times 9.8

14. Force equals mass times:
    a. Velocity
    b. Mass squared
    c. Acceleration
    d. Momentum

15. Work is defined as force times:
    a. Distance
    b. Energy
    c. Weight
    d. Joules

16. If an individual did 120 J of work in 2 seconds, how many W would that equal?
    a. 40
    b. 60
    c. 240
    D. 20

17. What type of energy does a boulder rolling down a mountain have?
    a. Chemical
    b. Potential
    c. Kinetic
    d. Nuclear

18. The potential energy of a boulder sitting on top of the Empire State Building is the same as:
    a. Its mass times its falling distance
    b. Two times its weight
    c. The kinetic energy stored
    d. The work needed to lift it there

19. Based on the law of conservation of energy, energy can never be:
    a. Regained
    b. Transferred
    c. Stored
    d. Destroyed

20. Mass times velocity is the formula for:
    a. Acceleration
    b. Work
    c. Force
    d. Momentum

Answer Key

Answers to Pretest

1. a

2. c

3. d

4. c

5. d

6. a

7. b

8. b

9. a

10. c

Answers to Review

1. Time, density

2. Derived

3. Density, specific gravity

4. Metric, meters, centimeters, millimeters (mm)

5. SI system, kilograms, seconds, degrees K, amperes (A)

6. Matter

7. Energy

8. Matter, protons, neutrons, and electrons

9. Mass, large, kilograms

10. Gravity

11. Inertia

12. Friction, force, inertia

13. Momentum, velocity

14. Momentum

15. Force, inertia, momentum or inertia

16. Gravity, mechanical force

17. Acceleration, positive acceleration, negative acceleration

18. Force, mass, acceleration

19. Newton, meter

20. Gravity

21. Work, distance, joule

22. Power, time, watt

23. Energy, energy, kinetic, potential

24. Energy, potential

Answers to Learning Quiz

1. The correct answer is 16. With 4 qt in a gal and 2 pt in a qt, there must be 8 pt in a gal. Thus there are 16 pt in 2 gal. Many of the equations used in physics are not much more complicated than the math in this question.

2. It will take 7 seconds. Whenever you are solving an equation with an unknown in it, you can perform any function to *both sides* of the equation to help solve it.

3. The answer is yes. The bottle would then have air in it, and air, like any gas, still has matter. You just can't see it because the tiny particles of matter are spread out in gasses. Everything consists of matter, regardless of whether you can see it or not. Only if we could somehow remove all the air molecules out of the bottle and obtain a perfect vacuum would the bottle truly be empty.

4. The answer is C. The weight doesn't change, because all the matter (and thus all the mass) is still present on the scale. The only thing that has changed is that the water was absorbed by the rice, and this entered the student's stomach. In both situations, the total mass of the student, the rice, the water, and the pan were on the scale.

5. The answer is 2. The original ball's momentum was 1×6, or 6 units. All 6 units went to the other two balls. The 1-kg ball moving at 2 m/sec has 2 of the units of momentum, meaning that the other 4 went to the 2-kg ball. Therefore it must also have a velocity of 2 m/sec to have a momentum of 4.

6. The answer is 259 J or, to be more precise, 258.72 J. It's a simple calculation. First, force is mass times acceleration, or 6 kg of books $\times$ 9.8 m/sec^2 gravity to overcome. Since work is force times distance, just multiply that answer by the total distance, which is 4.4.

7. In this case we know that there is no longer any mechanical energy present in the rock—neither potential nor kinetic energy. Therefore the energy must have been transformed into a different kind of energy. The kinetic energy of the boulder is transformed into heat, another form of energy. In any matter, regardless of whether it is a solid, liquid, or gas, the molecules have a natural movement, which causes kinetic energy. Heat is a measure of this kinetic energy. Making something warmer makes the molecules move more quickly than when the object is cooler.

    This is the reason why most substances expand when heated: the molecules move faster, pushing each other apart somewhat and enlarging the size of the object.

When the falling boulder strikes the ground, the impact jars the molecules of the ground, causing them to move faster and become warmer, creating kinetic energy. Hence there is conservation of energy.

Answers for Applications

1. The formula for velocity is: $v = d/t$. In this case the formula would read $v = 1000$ m/300 seconds, or velocity equals 3.333 m/sec.

2. The formula for momentum is mass times velocity. The mass of the man and his car are 1000 kg on earth and on the new planet, because mass does not change; weight does, because it is the result of gravity and mass. The momentum is then 1000 kg $\times$ 10 m/sec, or 10,000 kg-m/sec.

3. The formula for force is mass times acceleration. In this case the 1000 kg of mass 39.8 m/sec^2 = 9,800 newtons.

4. The force required to move the 1000-kg capstone is 9,800 newtons (1000 $\times$ 9.8). The work required to move it to the top is 9,800 times 300 m, or 2,940,000 J.

5. The force required to lift the box is 98 newtons. The work required to move it 10 m is 980 J. Since power is work divided by time, Joe uses 98 W on Monday and 196 W on Wednesday.

6. Knowing that the formula for momentum is $p = mv$, Joe should quickly determine that each object has a momentum of 50. Where Joe stands makes little difference.

Atomic Structure and Matter

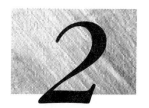

Self-Assessment Pretest

Use this pretest to assess your knowledge of the material in this module before you begin to work through the following exercises. Circle the best answer for each of the following questions. The answers are at the end of this module.

1. Helium, neon, and argon are not known to bond with any other gasses; as such they are called:
   a. Compound gasses
   b. Noble gasses
   c. Inert gasses

2. What is a hydrogen atom with one neutron called?
   a. Isomer
   b. Isobar
   c. Isotope
   d. Alpha particle

3. What is the atomic number of an atom with three protons, five neutrons, and five electrons?
   a. 3
   b. 5
   c. 8
   d. 13

4. Which of the following has the least mass?
   a. Proton
   b. Neutron
   c. Electron

5. An alpha particle is not an atom because it has no:
   a. Protons
   b. Electrons
   c. Energy
   d. Neutrons

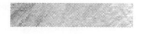

6. Which of the following are particles of energy that have no mass?
   a. Alpha rays
   b. Gamma rays
   c. Beta rays

the origin come from the nucleus

Gamma rays have highest frequency

Alpha most ionizing

X-ray most penetrating

Beta electron

7. What electrical charge do stable atoms have?
   a. Neutral
   b. Positive
   c. Negative

8. In stable atoms there are equal numbers of:
   a. Protons and neutrons
   b. Neutrons and photons
   c. Protons and photons
   d. Protons and electrons

9. During the process of decay a radioactive element emits:
   a. Particles of mass and energy
   b. Neutrons
   c. Electrons
   d. Protons

10. If an atom of a stable element loses one electron, its electrical charge will change to:
    a. Neutral
    b. Positive
    c. Negative

Key Terms

Before continuing, be sure you can define the following key terms.

Alpha particle: a particle that has two protons bound to two neutrons, but no electrons. This particle has the same nucleus as a helium atom, but an alpha particle is not an atom because it has no electrons.

AMU: the abbreviation for atomic mass unit (see definition below).

Atomic group: a grouping in the Periodic Table of the Elements that is determined by the number of electrons in the outermost electron shell of the atoms in each element.

Atomic mass: the total mass of an atom, measured by the mass of protons, neutrons, and electrons.

Atomic mass number: the number of protons plus the number of neutrons in the nucleus.

Atomic mass unit: the measurement unit based on the standard of the carbon-12 atom.

Atomic number: the number of protons in an atom.

Becquerel: the SI unit used to measure radioactive decay, defined as 1 decay event per second; abbreviated as Bq.

Beta particle: a tiny particle like an electron that forms inside an unstable nucleus. Because it has a negative charge, it is instantly ejected from the positively-charged nucleus. A beta particle is like an electron except that it did not originate in an electron shell.

Binding energy: the energy that holds protons and neutrons together in the nucleus through the force of attraction; the amount of energy needed to break up the nucleus.

Compound: a combination of elements bonded together. Compounds are very different from the elements that make them up because a compound is a whole new substance, not just a mix of its elements.

Covalent bonding: the process in which two atoms bond by sharing some of the same electrons, which revolve around both nuclei.

Curie: a measure of the rate of radioactive decay; the amount of material that has 370 billion nuclei decaying in 1 second; abbreviated as Ci.

Electromagnetic energy: pure energy, rather than particles with mass. The term is used because rays of electromagnetic energy have properties of both electrical energy and magnetic energy. Electromagnetic energy travels at the speed of light.

Electron: one of three fundamental units of an atom. An electron orbits around the nucleus of an atom and has very little mass. It has a negative electrical charge.

Electron affinity: the ability of the positively-charged atom's nucleus to attract electrons.

Electron binding energy: the energy that keeps electrons in their shells. The electron binding energy of any one electron depends on two factors: how close the electron is to the nucleus, and the total number of electrons in the atom.

Electron shell: the orbit of an electron that surrounds the nucleus of an atom.

Element: the simplest form of a substance that composes matter. Each element has only one unique type of atom in it, with a set number of protons. There are 92 elements existing in the natural world, and other elements have been created artificially.

Fundamental particle: a basic component of an atom, including the electron, neutron, and proton.

Half-life: the length of time it takes for half the atoms in a certain amount of an element to decay; the unit used to measure radioactivity.

Inert gas: a gas that is not known to bond with other elements to form a compound.

Ionic bonding: the process in which an electron transfers from one atom to another.

Ionization: the process of turning an atom into an ion by adding or removing an electron. In either case the change in the number of electrons changes the electrical charge of the atom.

Ionization energy: the amount of energy required to remove an electron from an atom.

Isobars: two atoms that have a different number of protons but the same total number of protons and neutrons and therefore the same atomic mass.

Isomers: atoms that have the same number of protons and neutrons but a different binding energy.

Isotones: atoms that have the same number of neutrons but a different number of protons.

Isotopes: atoms that have the same number of protons but a different number of neutrons.

Molecule: the smallest structure of combined atoms that can exist independently and retain the characteristics of the element or compound.

Negative ion: an atom that has an extra electron and therefore a negative charge.

Neutron: one of the three fundamental units of an atom. A neutron has the same atomic mass as a proton but has a neutral electrical charge.

Noble gas: a gas that does not easily react with other elements to form a compound.

Nucleus: the center of an atom; it consists of at least one proton. All elements except hydrogen have a nucleus that includes neutrons.

Period: a quality of elements in the periodic table. Atoms in each period have the same number of electron shells. There are seven periods that correspond to the seven electron shells.

Periodic Table of the Elements: The Periodic Table of the Elements shows the atomic number and the atomic mass of all the elements arranged in an orderly way.

Photon: a particle of energy that has no mass.

Positive ion: an atom that is short one electron and therefore has a positive charge because of the unpaired proton.

Proton: one of the three fundamental units of an atom. A proton has a positive electrical charge and is present in all atoms.

Radioactive decay: the process by which radionuclides (radioactive atoms) emit particles and energy.

Radioactive element: an element composed of atoms with unstable nuclei that radiates particles and energy.

Radioactivity: a general term for the processes by which atoms with unstable nuclei radiate excess energy in the form of particles and energy.

Radionuclide: a radioactive atom.

Stable atom: an atom that has the same number of protons and electrons.

Strong nuclear force: the force of attraction between all the particles of a nucleus, both protons and neutrons.

Topical Outline

The following material is covered in this module.

I. An atom is made up of three fundamental particles: the proton, neutron, and electron.
    A. The nucleus of an atom consists of at least one proton, and in all elements except hydrogen, at least one neutron.
        1. Protons are one of the three fundamental units of an atom and are present in the nuclei of all atoms. They have a positive electrical charge.
        2. Neutrons are one of the three fundamental units of an atom and, with the exception of hydrogen, are present in all elements. Neutrons have the same atomic mass as protons, but they have a neutral electrical charge.
        3. Binding energy holds protons and neutrons together in the nucleus through the force of attraction. It is also a measure of the amount of energy needed to break up the atom.
    B. Electron shells are the orbits of electrons surrounding the nucleus of an atom. There can be a maximum of seven electron shells around an atom.
        1. Electrons orbit the nucleus of an atom. In stable atoms there are equal numbers of electrons and protons. Electrons have very little mass and a negative electrical charge.
        2. Electron binding energy keeps electrons in their shells. The electron binding energy of any one electron depends on two factors: how close the electron is to the nucleus and the total number of electrons in the atom.
II. Elements are the simplest forms of substances that compose matter. Each element has only one unique type of atom in it, with a set number of protons. There are 92 elements existing in the natural world, and other elements have been created artificially.
III. Compounds are combinations of elements bonded together. Compounds are very different from the elements that make them up because a compound is an entirely different substance, not just a mix of its elements.
    A. Ionization is the process of turning an atom into an ion by adding or removing an electron. In either case the change in the number of electrons changes the electrical charge of the atom.
        1. Ionic bonding occurs when an electron transfers from one atom to another.
        2. Covalent bonding occurs when two atoms bond by sharing some of the same electrons, which revolve around both nuclei.
IV. Molecules are the smallest structures of combined atoms that can exist independently and retain the characteristics of the element or compound.

V. Radioactivity is a general term for the processes by which some unstable atoms emit excess energy in the form of particles and energy. Such particles and energy are said to radiate from the atom; hence the term *radiation*.
   A. Electromagnetic energy is pure energy rather than particles with mass. The term is used because rays of electromagnetic energy have properties of both electrical energy and magnetic energy. Electromagnetic energy travels at the speed of light.
   B. Alpha particles are emitted during radiation. They have two protons bound to two neutrons, but no electrons.
   C. Beta particles are tiny particles similar to electrons, except that they form inside the nucleus of an unstable atom. Because they have a negative charge, they are instantly ejected from the positively-charged nucleus.
   D. Photons are particles of energy that have no mass. Gamma rays are streams of photons.
   E. Half-life is the length of time it takes for half the atoms in an element to decay. It is used to measure radioactivity.
      1. A curie (Ci) is a measure of the rate of radioactive decay. It is also the amount of material that has 370 billion nuclei decaying in 1 second.
      2. Becquerel (Bq) is the SI unit used to measure radioactive decay. It is defined as 1 decay event per second.

Review

1. The basic structure of an atoms is one or more small _electron_ in orbit around a larger, denser _nucleus_. Like our solar system and the space between our sun and the planets, there is mostly empty space between the _electron_ and the nucleus.

2. The basic parts of an atom are electrons, neutrons, and protons. These are often called the _fundamental particles_ . The _protons_ and _neutrons_ together make up the nucleus, while electrons are contained in the _shells_ .

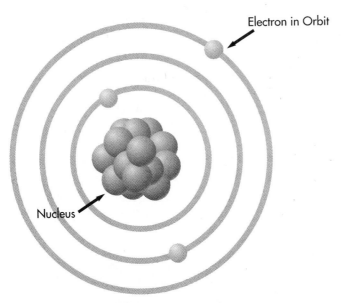

BOHR'S MODEL OF THE ATOM

3. Electromagnetic rays are pure energy, not particles with _mass_ . X-rays used in radiography are a form of _electromagnetic energy_

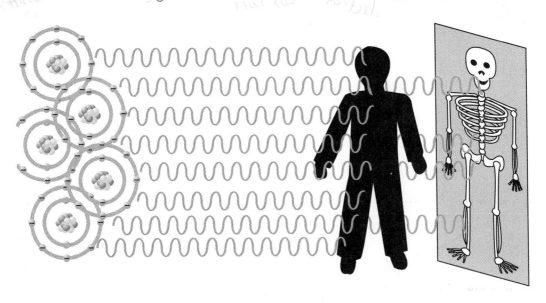

4. Although there is actually a tiny difference in the amount of _mass_ in protons and neutrons, each is said to have an _atomic_ number of 1. Unlike protons and neutrons, electrons have an atomic mass number of __0__ .

5. An important characteristic of atoms is the atomic number. This is the number of _protons_ in the nucleus. The _atomic mass_ is the total mass of the atom.

Fundamental particle	Atomic number	Atomic mass units (amu)	Mass in kilograms
Proton	1	1.00728	1.673×10^{-27}
Neutron	1	1.00867	1.675×10^{-27}
Electron	0	0.00055	9.11×10^{-31}

6. A special kind of chart called the _Periodic Table_ of the Elements shows the _atomic number_ and the atomic mass of all the elements arranged in an orderly way.

7. _Isotopes_ are atoms that have a different number of neutrons but the same number of _protons_.

8. _Isobars_ are atoms that have different numbers of protons but the same total number of protons and neutrons. Thus isobars have the same _atomic mass_.

9. _Isomers_ are atoms with the same number of protons and neutrons but different amounts of _energy_ within their nuclei because of differences in how those protons and _neutrons_ are arranged.

10. Atoms are _Isotones_ if they have the same number of neutrons but a different number of _protons_.

11. The nucleus of an atom is held together by the _binding force_. This is the term for the force of _attraction_ between all the particles of the _nucleus_, both protons and neutrons.

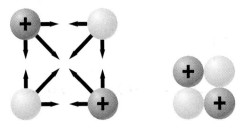

12. More neutrons are generally present in larger, heavier elements because the strong nuclear force they add to the nucleus is needed to help stabilize such _atoms_ to keep the _nucleus_ from breaking up.

13. The force that holds _protons_ and neutrons together in the nucleus is called the _binding force_. This is the sum of the strong nuclear forces that attract and thereby pull together the individual protons and _neutrons_ in the nucleus.

Periodic Table

Period	I	II													III	IV	V	VI	VII	VIII
1	1 H 1.00797																			2 He 4.0026
2	3 Li 6.939	4 Be 9.0122													5 B 10.811	6 C 12.01115	7 N 14.0067	8 O 15.9994	9 F 18.9984	10 Ne 20.183
3	11 Na 22.9898	12 Mg 24.312													13 Al 26.9815	14 Si 28.086	15 P 30.9738	16 S 32.064	17 Cl 35.453	18 A 39.948
4	19 K 39.102	20 Ca 40.08	21 Sc 44.956	22 Ti 47.90	23 V 50.924	24 Cr 51.996	25 Mn 54.9380	26 Fe 55.847	27 Co 58.9332	28 Ni 58.71	29 Cu 63.54	30 Zn 65.37			31 Ga 69.72	32 Ge 72.59	33 As 74.9216	34 Se 78.96	35 Br 79.909	36 Kr 83.80
5	37 Rb 85.47	38 Sr 87.62	39 Y 88.905	40 Zr 91.22	41 Nb 92.906	42 Mo 95.94	43 Tc [99]*	44 Ru 101.07	45 Rh 102.905	46 Pd 106.4	47 Ag 107.870	48 Cd 112.40			49 In 114.82	50 Sn 118.69	51 Sb 121.75	52 Te 127.60	53 I 126.9044	54 Xe 131.30
6	55 Cs 132.905	56 Ba 137.34	★ 57–71	72 Hf 178.49	73 Ta 180.948	74 W 183.85	75 Re 186.2	76 Os 190.2	77 Ir 192.2	78 Pt 195.09	79 Au 96.967	80 Hg 200.59			81 Tl 204.37	82 Pb 207.19	83 Bi 208.980	84 Po [210]*	85 At [210]*	86 Rn [222]*
7	87 Fr [223]*	88 Ra [226]*	+ 89–103																	

Group →
Period →

Inner Transition Metals:

★ Lanthanides

+ Actinides

14. In all stable atoms there are the same number of _electrons_ and _protons_ . The hydrogen atom

    has one of each, the helium atom has two of each, and so on.

15. Electrons were discovered with the development of the early _Cathode ray tube_ . An electric current pass-

    ing through certain gasses produced a glowing ray that could be deflected by a _magnetis_ , showing

    that it contained particles that were attracted by magnetic forces.

16. Each proton has a _positive charge_ , and each electron has a negative charge. Since there are the same

    number of both in a normal, stable atom, atoms normally have a _neutral charge_ because the negatives

    are balanced by the positives.

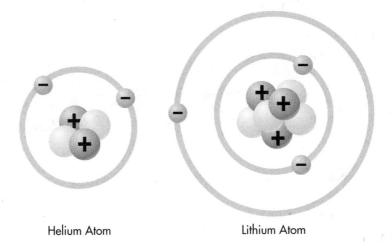

Helium Atom   Lithium Atom

17. The SI unit now used to measure the rate of radioactive decay is called the _Baqueral_ , which is

    defined as 1 decay event per _Second_ . One _curie_ measures the decay of 370 billion nuclei

    in 1 second.

18. The orbits of electrons are called ___electronic Shells___ because the electrons move in three dimensions all

around the ___nucleus___, not in flat two dimensions as often pictured. There are ___7___ shells in

the largest naturally occurring atom, uranium.

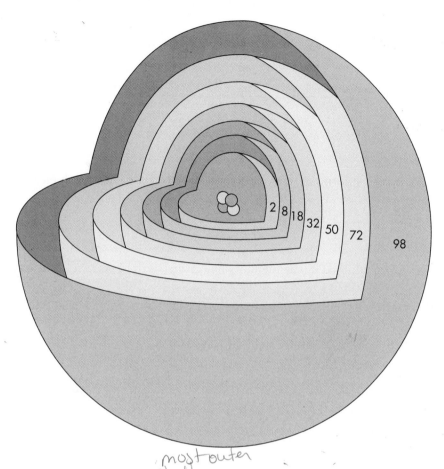

19. Only eight electrons can be in the ___most outer Shells___ of any atom, even though the same shell may hold

more electrons as long as it is not the outermost shell.

20. Electrons are kept in their shells in the atom by ___electron binding force___ . The amount of energy of any one

electron depends on two factors: how close it is to the ___nucleus___, and the total number of elec-

trons in the atom.

21. An atom with an extra electron has a ___negative charge___ because of that extra electron's negative charge.
This is called a ___negative ion___ .

22. An atom that is short one electron has a positive charge because of the positive charge of the one _proton_ that is not balanced by an electron. This is called a _ion_ [positive].

23. _Ionic bond_ occurs when an electron transfers from one atom to another. The atom losing the electron becomes a _ion_ [positive], and the atom gaining the electron becomes a _ion_ [negative].

24. In _bonding_ [covalent] two atoms are bonded by sharing some of the same electrons, which revolve around both _nuclei_.

25. Elements are the simplest forms of substances that compose _matter_. Each element has only one unique type of _atom_ in it, with a set number of _protons_.

26. Atomic groups are determined by the number of electrons in the _shell_ [outer most] of the atoms in each element. The atomic number is the number of _protons_ in the atom. The atomic mass is the actual mass of the _whole atom_ measured in atomic mass units.

27. Atoms in each period of the periodic table have the same number of _shells_ [electron], and there can only be _7_ periods.

28. Atoms can attract extra electrons because of a property called _affinity_ [electron]. A free electron passing by a hydrogen atom, for example, will be attracted to the _positive_ charge of the hydrogen atom's nucleus.

29. Radioactivity is a general term for the processes by which some _unstable_ atoms give off particles and _energy_. These emissions are said to _radiate_ from the atom; from this comes the term radiation.

30. Radioactivity involves the _nucleus_ of the atom, not the electrons. The movement of electrons creates an _electricity_ , not radiation. Radioactivity results from atoms with an unstable nucleus that contains too much _energy_ .γ

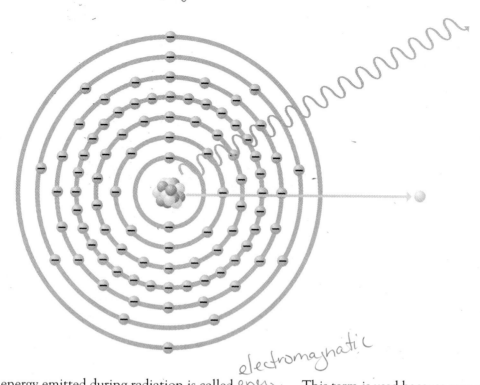

31. The energy emitted during radiation is called _energy_ (electromagnetic) . This term is used because rays of electro-magnetic energy have properties of both _electrical_ energy and _magnetic_ energy.

32. Alpha particles have a _positive_ charge. An alpha particle is two _protons_ bound to two neu-trons. An alpha particle is not an atom because it has no _electrons_ .

33. A beta particle is a tiny particle like an _electron_ that forms inside an unstable nucleus. It has a _negative_ charge; the nucleus has a _positive_ charge.

34. The rate at which a _radioactive_ substance decays is called a half-life. A half-life is the length of time it takes for half the _atoms_ in a certain amount of the element to decay.

Learning Quiz

The following material is similar to the interactive exercises found in the CD-ROM version of this module operated in the "student mode." These questions will allow you to review the concepts presented in this module and will help you to gain a more complete understanding of the material.

1. Is the following statement true or false? Since neutrons do not carry a charge, the number of neutrons in an isotope does not change the way an isotope behaves.

2. If a proton has a mass of 1.673×10^{-27} would the number be written by putting 27 zeros to the left or the right of the decimal point?

3. Based on what you have learned about what holds an atom together, what force must be overcome to release the energy of an atomic bomb? Remember, the words nuclear and nucleus are related.

4. As you learned in Module 1, the equation for kinetic energy is KE = ½ mv^2. Kinetic energy is half of the mass of the object times the square of its velocity. Although the atomic energy of electrons is not precisely the same, what should occur as the electrons in an atom move faster?

5. If you compared an atom to our planetary system, the sun would be the nucleus and the planets would be the electrons. Gravity is what keeps the planets from shooting off into outer space. What keeps the electrons from shooting out of the atom?

6. Consider two pairs of twins, one identical and one fraternal. Identical twins are very similar because they have exactly the same genes, as a result of one egg joined with one sperm. They share the same chromosomal makeup and often experience close bonds as a result. Fraternal twins, on the other hand, do not share exactly the same genes. However, by being so close together, they are often attracted to each other and develop bonds that are just as strong. Which type of twins resembles covalent bonding?

7. Why are atoms with only one electron in their outer shell more likely to become ions?

8. Why do the six noble gasses not easily react with other atoms to form compounds?

9. In the creation of a compound that mixed 2 parts nickel with 1 part lead, would the compound contain more atoms of the lead element or nickel element, or is there some other answer?

10. The atoms in most metals bond in a way that allows electrons to readily move throughout the bonded atoms. Why does this help electricity flow through metals?

11. We know that sunlight can knock electrons off atoms, and the electrons can then drift over to other atoms and form a compound. We also know that sunlight can cause cancer that develops years after exposure. What can sunlight do to a chromosome that can set off the process of chemical change?

Applications

1. You have heard the expression "opposites attract." This is true between negative and positive atoms and between starry-eyed lovers. However, in some cases starry-eyed lovers are not opposites and are attracted to each other because they share the same values. Which pair of starry-eyed lovers would best represent ionic bonding, those who share values or those who are opposites?

2. The basic parts of an atom are electrons, neutrons, and protons. These are often called the fundamental particles. If the hydrogen atom has an atomic number of 1 and an atomic mass of 1.00797, how many protons and neutrons make up the nucleus?

3. All atoms of sodium, symbolized Na, have 11 protons. The atomic mass of sodium in the Periodic Table of the Elements is 22.9898. If most sodium atoms have 12 neutrons, why is the atomic mass number slightly less than 23 rather than slightly more than 23?

4. While there is no set ratio of protons to neutrons in the nucleus of an atom, the Periodic Table of the Elements reveals general trends. In increasingly large atoms, why does the ratio of neutrons to protons generally increase?

5. Atoms normally have a neutral charge because the negatives are balanced by the positives. If an electron is added or removed, however, the atom would no longer have a neutral charge. What charge would an atom with an extra electron have?

6. Imagine two single atoms floating through space. By chance they come in contact, and a single electron from one atom transfers to the other atom. How would the changing electrical charge of the two atoms affect them, and what is this process called?

7. The Periodic Table of the Elements arranges the elements in a variety of ways. The element francium, which has an atomic number of 87, is in the first group and the seventh period of the chart. Based on this information, how many protons, electrons, and electron shells does francium have?

8. Sodium is a soft metal that is very poisonous, and chlorine is a yellow-green gas that is also very poisonous. When these two elements are combined to make a compound, why can we ingest them without suffering any ill effects?

9. Sound travels in waves as molecules that are vibrating pass that energy on to adjoining molecules that also vibrate and pass it on. Based on this, why would you not hear someone calling for help in outer space?

10. A helium atom is made up of two protons, two neutrons, and two electrons. What would the helium atom become if the two electrons were removed?

11. To help understand the concept of half-life, imagine 100 kg of radioactive material with a half-life of 100 years. After 400 years, how much of the material would have decayed? How many half lives would it take for all the material to decay?

Posttest

Circle the best answer for each of the following questions. Your instructor has the correct answers.

1. Which of the following is not a fundamental particle?
   a. Proton
   b. Neutron
   c. Electron
   d. Alpha particle

2. What fundamental particle has an atomic mass number of 0?
   a. Electron
   b. Neutron
   c. Proton
   d. Alpha particle

3. The atomic number of an element is the number of:
   a. Electrons in the nucleus
   b. Protons in the nucleus
   c. Neutrons in the nucleus

4. Atomic mass is measured by the:
   a. Number of protons
   b. Number of neutrons
   c. Number of electrons
   d. Sum of protons, electrons, and neutrons

5. Neutrons play an important role in adding stability to:
   a. Protons
   b. Electrons
   c. The nucleus
   d. Isotopes

6. What are atoms called that have a different number of neutrons but the same number of protons?
   a. Isotopes
   b. Isobars
   c. Isomers
   d. Isotones

7. What are atoms called that have the same number of neutrons but a different number of protons?
   a. Isotopes
   b. Isobars
   c. Isomers
   d. Isotones

8. What are atoms called that have the same number of neutrons and protons but different binding energy?
   a. Isotopes
   b. Isobars
   c. Isomers
   d. Isotones

9. What holds the nucleus of an atom together?
   a. Isotopes
   b. Strong nuclear force
   c. Electron shell
   d. Electron binding energy

10. Binding energy is the amount of energy needed to:
    a. Create an isomer
    b. Break up a nucleus
    c. Split a neutron

11. What is the maximum number of electrons shells possible in an atom?
    a. 7
    b. 9
    c. 14
    d. 21

12. All stable atoms have the same number of:
    a. Protons and neutrons
    b. Neutrons and electrons
    c. Protons and electrons

13. What charge does an atom normally have?
    a. Positive
    b. Negative
    c. Neutral

14. The outermost shell of an atom can have a maximum of:
    a. 8 electrons
    b. 39 electrons
    c. 14 electrons

15. What keeps electrons in the shells of their atoms?
    a. Strong nuclear force
    b. Electron binding energy
    c. Neutrons

16. What electrical charge does an atom with an extra electron have?
    a. Positive
    b. Negative
    c. Neutral

17. What electrical charge does an atom that is short one electron have?
    a. Positive
    b. Negative
    c. Neutral

18. Through the process of ionic bonding, two atoms:
    a. Split
    b. Attract
    c. Repel

19. What is the process called in which two atoms bond by sharing some of the same electrons?
    a. Ionic bonding
    b. Covalent bonding
    c. Electron binding

20. Each element has only one unique type of atom in it with a set number of:
    a. Protons
    b. Neutrons
    c. Photons

21. Atoms that have eight electrons in their outermost electron shell:
    a. Tend to be unstable and combine with other atoms
    b. Are likely to form ions
    c. Are less likely to form ions that combine with other atoms

22. Atoms in each period of the Periodic Table of the Elements have the same number of:
    a. Protons
    b. Electrons
    c. Neutrons
    d. Electron shells

23. What are combinations of elements that are bonded together called?
    a. Isobars
    b. Isotopes
    c. Compounds
    d. Ions

24. In the process of radioactive decay, particles and energy are radiated from:
    a. The nucleus
    b. The electron shell
    c. Ions
    d. Isotopes

25. Emission of particles and energy during the process of radiation is called:
    a. Nuclear energy
    b. Electromagnetic energy
    c. Strong magnetic force

26. Photons are emitted in:
    a. Alpha rays
    b. Gamma rays
    c. Beta rays
    d. All of the above

27. What is the particle called that is made of two protons bound to two neutrons?
    a. Photon
    b. Beta particle
    c. Alpha particle
    d. Gamma particle

28. What is the electrical charge of beta particles?
    a. Positive
    b. Negative
    c. Neutral
    d. Changing

29. The SI unit used to measure 1 decay event per second is called:
    a. Half-life
    b. Ci
    c. Bq

30. The nucleus of every atom has at least one:
    a. Electron
    b. Proton
    c. Neutron

Answer Key

Answers to Pretest

1. c

2. c

3. a

4. c

5. b

6. b

7. a

8. d

9. a

10. b

Answers to Review

1. Electrons, nucleus, electrons

2. Fundamental particles, protons, neutrons, electron shells

3. Mass, electromagnetic energy

4. Mass, atomic mass, 0

5. Protons, atomic mass

6. Periodic Table, atomic number

7. Isotopes, protons

8. Isobars, atomic mass number

9. Isomers, energy, neutrons

10. Isotones, protons

11. Strong nuclear force or binding energy, attraction, nucleus

12. Atoms, nucleus

13. Protons, binding energy, neutrons

14. Electrons, protons

15. Cathode ray tube, magnet

16. Positive charge, neutral charge

17. Bq, second, Ci

18. Electron shells, nucleus, seven

19. Outermost shell

20. Electron binding energy, nucleus

21. Negative charge, negative ion

22. Proton, positive ion

23. Ionic bonding, positive ion, negative ion

24. Covalent bonding, nuclei

25. Matter, atom, protons

26. Outermost electron shell, protons, whole atom

27. Electron shells, seven

28. Electron affinity, positive

29. Unstable, energy, radiate

30. Nucleus, electric current, energy

31. Electromagnetic energy, electrical, magnetic

32. Positive, protons, electrons

33. Electron, negative, positive

34. Radioactive, atoms

Answers to Learning Quiz

1. False. Neutrons add stability to atoms. Isotopes of the same atoms can behave very differently.

2. To the left of the decimal point. A positive number of 1.673×10^{27} would place the decimal point to the right of the 27 zeros and would represent millions of kilograms. In this case the negative number moves the decimal point to the left of the 27 zeros.

3. Binding energy. A nuclear bomb occurs by splitting the nucleus of an atom. It is the binding energy that holds the nucleus together and must be overcome.

4. The amount of energy in the atom increases. Just as the kinetic energy of a car increases as its speed increases, the energy of an atom increases as the speed of the electrons increases.

5. Electron binding energy. Two factors determine the amount of electron binding energy: how close the electron is to the nucleus, and the number of electrons in the atom. Most of the binding energy comes from the force of attraction between the negatively-charged electrons and the positively-charged protons.

6. Identical twins. Just as identical twins share the same genes, covalent bonding occurs when atoms share the same electrons.

7. Because there is room in that shell for other electrons to be added. It is also easier to knock that one electron out of its shell than it would be to knock an electron out of a more stable atom with a full electron shell.

8. Each of these gasses has eight electrons in its outermost electron shell. Since the most electrons an outermost shell can contain is eight, the shells are "full." Thus these gasses tend to be very stable and much less likely to form ions that combine with other atoms.

9. Neither of the elements would be present in a compound. While compounds are made from elements, they are very different from the elements that make them up because a compound is a whole new substance, not just a mix of its elements.

10. Because an electric current is a flow of electrons.

11. Just as sunlight can move electrons in the air, it can penetrate the skin and knock an electron from a molecule that forms part of a chromosome. This then sets off the process of chemical change that years from now can lead to skin cancer.

Answers to Applications

1. Those who are opposites. Ionic bonding occurs when two atoms are attracted to each other because of their opposite charges. Covalent bonding occurs when atoms share the same electrons.

2. Hydrogen is the only element that does not have any neutrons. It has one proton and one electron.

3. Sodium is an isotope, atoms that have a different number of neutrons but the same number of protons. The atomic mass of sodium is an average of sodium atoms that have 12 neutrons and those that have 11 neutrons.

4. More neutrons are generally present in larger, heavier elements because the strong nuclear force they add to the nucleus is needed to help stabilize such atoms and to keep the nucleus from breaking up.

5. A negative charge would occur because the addition of an electron would shift the balance of the atom from neutral to negative. This is called a negative ion.

6. The atom losing an electron would become positively charged and the atom gaining an electron would become negatively charged. Since opposites attract, the two atoms would be held to each other by ionic bonding.

7. The atomic number 87 means that there are 87 protons in the atom. The first group consists of atoms with only a single electron in the outermost electron shell. The seventh period consists of atoms with seven electron shells.

8. The compound of sodium and chlorine is called sodium chloride or salt. When two or more elements form a compound, that compound is not just a mix of the elements but an entirely new substance. In this case the two poisons become salt.

9. Sound depends on matter to pass from one place to another. Since space is a vacuum with little or no matter, sound cannot travel there.

10. An alpha particle, which consists of two protons and two neutrons but no electrons.

11. At the end of 400 years the material would have decayed through 4 half-lives with 6.25 kg of the material remaining. As for complete decay, with radioactive elements and trillions of atoms present, the radiation lasts almost forever—or until the last atom decays.

Electromagnetic Radiation

Self-Assessment Pretest

Use this pretest to assess your knowledge of the material in this module before you begin to work through the following exercises. Circle the best answer for each of the following questions. The answers are at the end of this module.

1. How is a hertz (Hz) defined?
   a. 1000 cycles per second
   b. By the number of cycles in the red spectrum of light
   c. By the rate of decay of a single photon
   d. 1 cycle per second

2. The bending of light rays through a prism is called:
   a. Deflection
   b. Refraction
   c. Absorption

3. Which of the following have photons?
   a. X-rays
   b. Gamma rays
   c. Visible light
   d. All of the above

4. Which of the following is true of all electromagnetic energy?
   a. It has photons
   b. It has varying levels of energy
   c. It moves at the speed of light
   d. All of the above

5. Frequency is determined by:
   a. The number of waves in 1 second
   b. The amplitude of the waves
   c. Inverse square law
   d. All of the above

6. Which of the following has the longest wavelength?
    a. AM radio
    b. FM radio
    c. Infrared light
    d. Visible light

7. Frequency rises as the:
    a. Wavelength shortens
    b. Wavelength becomes more unstable
    c. Wavelength moves slower
    d. Cycles grow longer

8. What does frequency times wavelength equal?
    a. Amplitude
    b. Velocity
    c. Hertz
    d. Cycle

9. What is the SI unit of measurement for frequency?
    a. Electron volt
    b. Cycle
    c. Hertz

10. Gamma rays originate in:
    a. The nucleus
    b. Protons
    c. Electron shells
    d. Alpha particles

Key Terms

Before continuing, be sure you can define the following key terms.

Absorbed: the condition of light when the light photons are stopped by a substance.

Alpha particle: a particle that has two protons and two neutrons bound together, but no electrons.

Amplitude: the height of a wave. A wave with a large amplitude is generally stronger than a wave with a small amplitude.

Attenuated: the condition of light when some of the photons are absorbed but some are transmitted through a substance.

De-excitation: the condition that occurs when an excited atom returns to its normal stable state. The electron that had jumped returns to its normal lower shell. Because the electron has a lower energy level in the lower shell, it must release the higher energy that made it excited. The released energy is a photon of light energy.

Electromagnetic energy: pure energy, rather than particles with mass. The term is used because rays of electromagnetic energy have properties of both electrical energy and magnetic energy. Electromagnetic energy travels at the speed of light.

Electromagnetic field: a field created by the vibrations of electromagnetic energy.

Electromagnetic spectrum: the range of electromagnetic energy in wavelengths. It is a continuum of every possible frequency. Radio waves, light, and x-rays are all terms for different ranges of wavelengths on this spectrum.

Energy: the ability to do work or make something happen. It can take the form of mechanical energy, heat, light, or electrical energy and is measured in the SI unit called the joule (J).

Energy vibration: a similar phenomenon to sound vibration, except the energy itself is vibrating, not the air molecules.

Excited: the state of an atom when something makes an electron jump to a higher shell. An excited atom has a higher energy level.

Frequency: the number of waves that go by in a second.

Gamma ray: a type of electromagnetic radiation at the high end of the spectrum with a frequency greater than visible light and ultraviolet light. Gamma rays originate in the nuclei of atoms that are decaying and, in the process, giving off alpha particles and a photon of energy.

Hertz: the SI unit of measurement for frequency (abbreviated Hz); 1 Hz is defined as 1 cycle per second.

Infrared light: a type of heat radiation; the infrared light in sunlight, for example, is what makes the sunlight feel warm upon one's skin.

Inverse square law: the principle that the intensity of light diminishes by a factor of the square of the distance from its source.

Ionizing radiation: the power to change atoms and thereby molecules inside a substance through contact; examples are x-rays and gamma rays.

Kilohertz: the frequency range in thousands of cycles per second; abbreviated as kHz.

Kinetic energy: the energy of an object in motion; abbreviated as KE.

Light: the electromagnetic energy in a certain range of wavelengths in the electromagnetic spectrum. It includes visible light, infrared light, and ultraviolet light.

Megahertz: the frequency range in millions of cycles per second; abbreviated as MHz.

Opaque: the property of a substance that totally absorbs light rays.

Photon: a particle of energy that has no mass; emitted as light or another form of electromagnetic energy.

Radiolucent: the property of a substance that allows x-rays to partially pass through it.

Radiopaque: the property of a substance that does not allow x-rays to pass through.

Refraction: the "bending" of light photons as they pass through one clear medium to another. The amount of refraction varies, depending on wavelength.

Roentgenogram: another term for radiograph.

Sine wave: the wave form of electromagnetic energy, the wave having regular characteristics such as a constant amplitude and wavelength.

Spectrum: a continuum of visible light that includes the frequency ranges of the various colors. Each color of the spectrum, as in a prism or rainbow, is a different frequency.

Speed of light: approximately 3×10^8 m/sec, or 300 million meters per second. All electromagnetic radiation travels at the same velocity through space, the speed of light.

Translucent: the property of a substance that partially absorbs, or attenuates, light rays.

Transmitted: the state of light photons that have passed through a substance such as air, clear glass, or the near vacuum of space.

Ultraviolet light: energy at a higher frequency that can interact with molecules in one's skin and cause sunburn or, over a long term, skin cancer.

Velocity: the speed at which an object is moving. It is measured by determining the distance an object travels in a specific period of time. Waves in the electromagnetic spectrum all travel at the same velocity, the speed of light, or 300 million meters per second.

Visible light: the range of light that humans can see; the total range of visible light is less than a millionth of 1% of the electromagnetic spectrum. The frequencies above and below visible light, ultraviolet and infrared, are still considered light because they share other characteristics with visible light.

Wave: a property of energy created by the vibrations of photons. It can be compared to a ripple that moves water molecules up and down on the surface of a pond.

Wavelength: the length of one wave, measured from the top of one wave to the top of the next. To calculate wavelength, divide the velocity (300 million meters per second) by the frequency.

X-rays: the result of a fast-moving electron striking the atoms of certain metals. X-rays are not emitted naturally from atoms but are produced when kinetic energy outside the atom excites the electrons. X-rays are similar to gamma rays except that they originate in the electron shells of atoms rather than in the nucleus.

Topical Outline

The following material is covered in this module.

I. The electromagnetic spectrum is the range of electromagnetic energy in wavelengths. It is a continuum of every possible frequency. Radio waves, light, and x-rays are all terms for different ranges of wavelengths on this spectrum.
    A. Electromagnetic energy is pure energy, rather than particles with mass. The term is used because rays of electromagnetic energy have properties of both electrical energy and magnetic energy. Electromagnetic energy travels at the speed of light.
    B. Velocity is measured by determining the distance an object travels in a specific period of time. Waves in the electromagnetic spectrum all travel at the same velocity, the speed of light, or 300 million m/sec.
    C. Wavelength is the length of one wave, measured from the top of one wave to the top of the next. To calculate wavelength, divide the velocity (300 million m/sec) by the frequency.
    D. Frequency refers to the number of waves that go by in a second.
       1. Hertz (Hz) is the SI unit of measurement for frequency. One Hz is defined as one cycle per second.

II. Light is the electromagnetic energy in a certain range of wavelengths in the electromagnetic spectrum. It includes visible light, infrared light, and ultraviolet light.
    A. Excitation of an atom occurs when something makes an electron jump to a higher shell. An excited atom has a higher energy level. De-excitation occurs when an excited atom returns to its normal stable state. The electron that has jumped thus falls back into its normal lower shell.
    B. A wave of energy is created by the vibrations of photons. It can be compared to a ripple that moves water molecules up and down on the surface of a pond.
    C. Photons are a stream of particles of energy emitted as light or other electromagnetic energy.
       1. Absorption occurs when light photons are stopped by a substance.
       2. Attenuation occurs when some photons are absorbed by a substance and some are transmitted through the substance.
    D. The inverse square law states that the intensity of light diminishes by a factor of the square of the distance from its source.

III. X-rays and gamma rays are similar, but the photons of gamma rays originate in the nucleus and the photons of x-rays originate in the electron shell. While gamma rays naturally occur in radioactive decay, x-rays are produced when kinetic energy outside the atom excites the electrons.

A. X-rays and gamma rays are called ionizing radiation because they have the power to change atoms and thereby molecules inside substances they strike.

Review

1. The illustration below shows seven molecules in a row labeled A through G. They represent the wave created by a pebble hitting water. As the _Kenitic_ energy moves out from the point of impact, molecule A is lifted first, then B. As the _wave_ continues, each molecule in turn rises. Then each falls again as the energy passes on and _gravity_ pulls it back down.

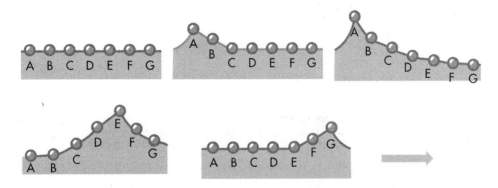

ENERGY WAVE MOVING MOLECULES IN SUCCESSION

2. Electromagnetic energy is similar to sound vibrations, but it is the _energy_ itself that is vibrating, not an ear drum or air molecules. The thing that is vibrating is actually an electromagnetic _wave field_.

3. Electromagnetic energy in a _vacuum_ would normally travel in a straight line. It can, however, be deflected by a _electric_ or _magnetic_ field. It may also be bent, or _refracted_, if it passes through a medium such as glass.

4. The _amplitude_ is the height of the wave. A wave with a large amplitude is generally _stronger_ than a wave with a small amplitude.

5. An important characteristic of light waves, and all electromagnetic energy, is wavelength. This is the _length_ of one wave, measured from the top of one wave to the _top_ of the next. There are very short waves in light. For instance, there are four to seven million _wavelengths_ of light in one _meter_ .

6. Both sound and energy have different _frequencies_ that are perceivable by different species. The human ear has a certain frequency range within which we can hear sounds. Dogs can hear certain _high frequency_ sounds that we cannot hear. Rattlesnakes and other pit vipers have special sensors by which to perceive heat radiated from nearby objects. Although they aren't quite "seeing" this _infrared_ energy, they are able to sense it in a way we cannot.

7. One of the great discoveries of modern physics, by James Maxwell in the second half of the 19th century, was that all waves of _electromagnetic_ energy travel at the same speed—the _speed of light_ . This was part of a larger discovery, that in fact all electromagnetic energy is very similar: it all has no _mass_ , carries energy in _waves_ , and moves at the speed of light.

8. In mathematics the wave form of electromagnetic energy is called a _sine wave_ . That means the wave has a regular shape with regular characteristics, such as a constant _wavelength_ and _amplitude_ .

9. The range in wavelengths is called the electromagnetic _spectrum_ . There is a continuum from one frequency to the next, with every possible _frequency_ existing here. Light, radio waves, and x-rays are all just terms for different ranges of _wave lengths_ in this spectrum.

10. Since all electromagnetic energy waves move at the same speed, there is a simple relationship between wavelength and _frequency_ . The longer the wavelength, the _lower_ the frequency of waves per second. The shorter the _wavelength_ , the higher the frequency. The SI unit of measurement for frequency is the _hertz_ .

11. All electromagnetic radiation travels at the same _~~speed~~ velocity_ , the speed of light, or 3×10^8 _meter_ per second. That means that with a wavelength of 1 m, 300 million _waves_ would pass by in 1 second.

12. Light is simply electromagnetic _energy_ in a certain range of wavelengths in the electromagnetic _spectrum_. In the illustration below, the range of visible light in the spectrum has been enlarged so it shows up. In reality, the total range of _visible_ light is less than a millionth of 1% of the _electromagnetic_ spectrum.

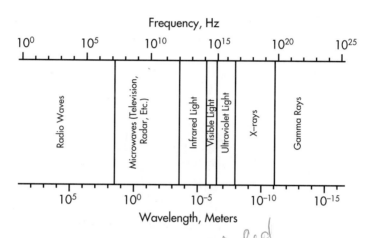

Frequency, Hz

10^0 10^5 10^{10} 10^{15} 10^{20} 10^{25}

Radio Waves

Microwaves (Television, Radar, Etc.)

Infrared Light

Visible Light

Ultraviolet Light

X-rays

Gamma Rays

10^5 10^0 10^{-5} 10^{-10} 10^{-15}

Wavelength, Meters

13. In addition to visible light, sunlight also contains _infrared_ light and ultraviolet light, which cannot be seen by the human eye. Infrared light is a type of _heat_ radiation—the infrared light in sunlight is what makes the sunlight feel warm upon one's skin. _Ultraviolet_ light is energy at a higher frequency that can interact with _molecules_ in one's skin and cause sunburn or, over a long term, skin cancer.

14. The eye can see the difference between green light and blue light because waves of _electromagnetic_

energy at different frequencies have different amounts of _energy_. The photons at different

frequencies have somewhat different characteristics. It is analogous to the nerves of one's hand

being able to feel the difference between pebbles and ice pellets dropped upon it at the same

speed. If they have the same mass and _velocity_, they both strike with the same momentum—

but a hand is able to feel the difference in temperature.

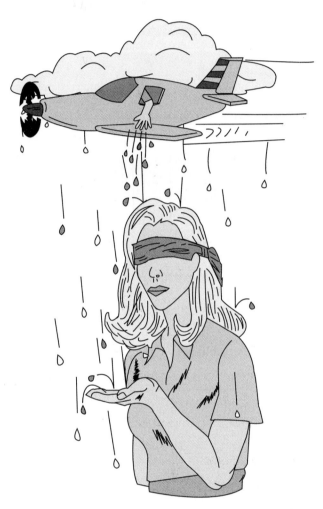

15. An atom does stay excited very long but returns to its normal _stable_ state. In doing so, the

electron that had been pushed into a higher electron shell falls back into its normal lower shell.

In the lower _shell_ it has a lower energy level, so it must release the higher _energy_ that

made it excited.

16. Light photons that pass through a substance such as air, clear glass, or the near vacuum of space are said to be _transmitted_. If the light photons are stopped by the substance, the light is said to be _absorbed_. If some of the photons are absorbed but some are transmitted through, the light is said to be _attenuated_.

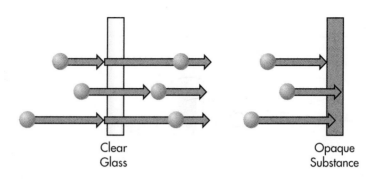

Clear
Glass

Opaque
Substance

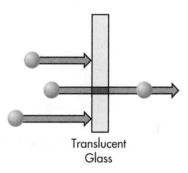

Translucent
Glass

17. The intensity of light is related to the number of waves or _particles_ emitted from the source, as well as the _distance_ of that source. Bright light has more photons than dim light, even though all these _photons_ may be at the same frequency, and each individual photon has the same amount of _energy_ as any other photon.

18. The figure below gives the equation for the inverse square law. To understand the inverse square law, it is helpful to remember that light also acts as _particle_. Even though photons are steadily emitted by the light source, as an object moves farther away from the source, fewer _photon_ will reach it. They are spreading out as they travel out in a wider area away from the _source_.

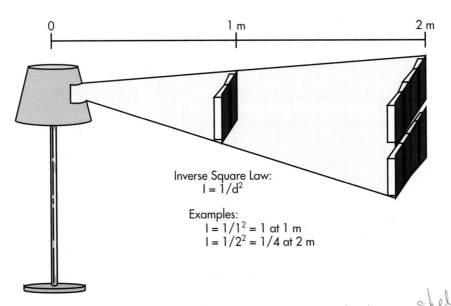

0   1 m   2 m

Inverse Square Law:
$I = 1/d^2$

Examples:
$I = 1/1^2 = 1$ at 1 m
$I = 1/2^2 = 1/4$ at 2 m

19. X-rays are similar to gamma rays except that they originate in the _electron shells_ of atoms rather than in the _nucleus_. Gamma rays occur naturally in _radioactive_ elements. X-rays, on the other hand, are not emitted naturally from atoms but are produced when _kinetic_ energy outside the atom excites the electrons.

Magenta is the color of the caution sign
of the radiation sign.

20. The figure below shows that x-rays have certain properties similar to _light_ that make them useful. They can be transmitted through certain substances, they are attenuated by other substances, such as _radiolucent_ soft tissues of the body, and they are absorbed by still other substances, such as bone or metals. No x-rays pass through the _radiopaque_ coin stuck in this person's throat.

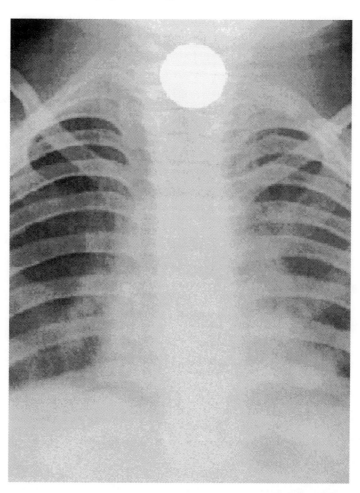

21. The amount of energy a photon has is proportional to its _frequency_. X-rays are not all at the same frequency, just as visible light covers a range on the _electromagnetic_ spectrum. The relationship between energy and frequency is the same for all photons. One photon at a frequency twice that of a second photon also has _2X_ as much energy. The equation for calculating the energy in _electron volts_ is: E (energy) = h (Planck's constant) × frequency (in Hz).

Learning Quiz

The following material is similar to the interactive exercises found in the CD-ROM version of this module operated in the "student mode." These questions will allow you to review the concepts presented in this module and will help you to gain a more complete understanding of the material.

1. What will happen to the direction of electromagnetic energy if it interacts with a magnetic or electric field?

2. What occurs to electromagnetic energy in the form of sunlight as it passes through a prism?

3. Why does the spectrum of colors in a rainbow or prism not begin and end abruptly, but rather slowly merge from one color into another?

4. What makes an electron jump to a higher electron shell and what happens when the electron returns to its normal state?

5. In the process of creating light in a light bulb, millions of electrons become excited and de-excited. What else is happening to make the light we see?

6. Why is there increased danger when radiation damages an individual's reproductive organs?

7. Why is lead used as a shield against x-rays?

Applications

1. Explain what occurs when a wave is described as having a frequency of 6 Hz, or cycles per second.

2. With a wavelength of 1 m, how many waves would pass by in 1 second if the frequency was 300 MHz?

3. Here is another quick problem to solve with frequency. If you know the velocity of a wave is the speed of light, or 3×10^8 m/sec, and the frequency is 3×10^{16} Hz, what is the wavelength?

4. Imagine yourself at a party when someone happens to mention that the wavelength of the color violet is 4×10^{-7} m. Not to be outdone, you quickly calculate the frequency of the color violet. Your boss, who is standing behind you, is amazed and gives you a promotion. What is the frequency of the color violet?

5. Is a photon of light emitted during the excitation process when an electron jumps to a higher shell or is a photon of light emitted during the de-excitation process when the atom returns to its normal state?

6. Imagine that you are a spy standing on a street corner holding an important document. At the same time, your rival is desperately trying to read the document by the light of a window sign 1 m away. You quickly calculate that, to prevent the document from being read, you will need to reduce the intensity of the light on the document by a factor of 1/9. How far away will you have to move?

Posttest

Circle the best answer for each of the following questions. Your instructor has the correct answers.

1. In electromagnetic energy, what is vibrating?
   a. Molecules
   b. Atoms
   c. Energy itself
   d. Alpha particles

2. Electromagnetic energy is a combination of:
   a. Beta and gamma rays
   b. Alpha and gamma rays
   c. Electric and magnetic fields

3. Electromagnetic energy in a vacuum would normally:
   a. Travel in a straight line
   b. Curve due to gravity
   c. Be deflected by matter
   d. Dissipate because of the lack of matter

4. A characteristic of photons is that they all have:
   a. Alpha particles
   b. Protons
   c. Electrons
   d. No mass

5. The height of a wave is called:
   a. Frequency
   b. Wavelength
   c. Amplitude
   d. Cycle

6. The measurement from the top of one wave to the top of the next is called:
   a. Frequency
   b. Wavelength
   c. Amplitude
   d. Cycle

7. Which of the following is *not* true of all electromagnetic energy?
   a. It has no mass
   b. It travels in waves
   c. It has a constant frequency
   d. It moves at the speed of light

8. The number of waves that go by in 1 second is called:
   a. Frequency
   b. Wavelength
   c. Amplitude

9. What is the frequency of a wave if only one-tenth of it goes by in 1 second?
   a. 1 cycle
   b. 10 cycles
   c. 0.10 cycle
   d. 100 cycles

10. Which of the following has the shortest wavelength?
   a. AM radio
   b. FM radio
   c. Infrared light
   d. Visible light

11. What is the range of wavelengths called that includes x-rays, radio waves, and visible light?
    a. Electromagnetic spectrum
    b. Frequency spectrum
    c. Range spectrum
    d. Energy spectrum

12. The longer the wavelength:
    a. The faster the wave moves
    b. The slower the wave moves
    c. The lower the frequency
    d. The higher the frequency

13. Which of the following is the speed of light?
    a. 3 million m/sec
    b. 30 million m/sec
    c. 300 million m/sec
    d. 3000 million m/sec

14. If a wavelength of electromagnetic energy is ½ m, what is the frequency?
    a. 150 MHz
    b. 600 MHz
    c. 75 MHz
    d. 300 MHz

15. What does velocity divided by frequency equal?
    a. Amplitude
    b. Wavelength
    c. Hz

16. The amount of energy carried in a wave increases as the:
    a. Frequency decreases
    b. Frequency increases
    c. Speed increases
    d. Speed decreases

17. Which of the following has the highest frequency?
    a. Visible light
    b. Infrared light
    c. Ultraviolet light

18. Which of the following is said to cause skin cancer?
    a. Visible light
    b. Infrared light
    c. Ultraviolet light

19. The bending of light rays through a prism is called:
    a. Deflection
    b. Refraction
    c. Absorption

20. What happens when an electron falls back into its normal lower shell?
    a. It emits energy
    b. A photon is released
    c. The atom returns to its normal state
    d. All of the above

21. If light photons are stopped by a substance, the light is said to be:
    a. Attenuated
    b. Absorbed
    c. Refracted
    d. Dispersed

22. Photoelectric cells convert sunlight into electricity when struck by a steady stream of:
    a. Beta particles
    b. Protons
    c. Photons
    d. Electrons

23. Based upon the inverse square law, how will the intensity of light change as the distance increases from 1 m to 4 m from the source?
    a. 1/16 as intense
    b. 1/4 as intense
    c. 1/2 as intense
    d. No change in intensity

24. As an unstable atom of a radioactive element naturally decays into a more stable state, it emits at that moment of decay a photon of energy and:
    a. An electron
    b. Two protons and two neutrons
    c. Two protons
    d. An electron and two protons

25. As photons collide with body tissue, what part of body atoms can be broken from molecules?
    a. Electrons
    b. Photons
    c. Alpha particles
    d. Neutrons

26. X-rays originate in:
    a. The nucleus
    b. Protons
    c. Electron shells
    d. Gamma rays

27. X-rays are generally attenuated by (choose *one* answer):
    a. Soft tissue
    b. Bones
    c. Metal
    d. Radiographic film

28. X-rays cannot pass through lead because it is:
    a. Radiolucent
    b. Opaque
    c. Translucent
    d. Radiopaque

29. X-rays and gamma rays are different from light because they have:
    a. Photons
    b. Enough energy to knock electrons out of atoms
    c. Electrons
    d. No mass

30. X-rays can have differing amounts of energy because the amount of energy a photon has is proportional to its:
    a. Atomic mass
    b. Amplitude
    c. Sine wave
    d. Frequency

31. What occurs when something makes an electron jump to a higher shell?
    a. It becomes a photon
    b. It loses energy
    c. It gains energy
    d. There is no change in energy

Answer Key

Answers to Pretest

1. d

2. b

3. d

4. d

5. a

6. a

7. a

8. b

9. c

10. a

Answers to Review

1. Kinetic, wave, gravity

2. Energy, wave

3. Vacuum, magnetic, electric, refracted

4. Amplitude, stronger

5. Length, top, wavelengths, meter (m)

6. Frequencies, high-frequency, infrared

7. Electromagnetic, speed of light, mass, waves

8. Sine wave, amplitude, wavelength

9. Spectrum, frequency, wavelengths

10. Frequency, lower, wavelength, Hz

11. Velocity, meters, waves

12. Energy, spectrum, visible, electromagnetic

13. Infrared, heat, Ultraviolet, molecules

14. Electromagnetic, energy, frequencies, velocity

15. Stable, electron, shell, energy

16. Transmitted, absorbed, attenuated

17. Particles, distance, photons, energy

18. Particles, photons, source

19. Electron shells, nucleus, radioactive, kinetic

20. Light, radiolucent, radiopaque

21. Frequency, electromagnetic, twice, electron-volts

Answers to Learning Quiz

1. Both magnetic and electric fields can cause electromagnetic energy to deflect from its normally straight-line course.

2. The sunlight is refracted. The colors of the prism correspond to the different frequencies that make up the visible light spectrum.

3. The word *spectrum* means that the array of energy types is continuous, one type merging into the next, rather than there being a set number of discrete types of energy. Take a good look at a rainbow. Even though there are separate colors, each color band gradually blends into the colors on both sides, without definite borders in between. That is how different kinds of electromagnetic energy work.

4. Energy is required to make an electron jump to a higher state. When the electron returns to its normal state it gives off energy, because it has a lower energy level in the lower shell.

5. Each jump of an electron produces a photon, and millions of these photons together produce light that is bright enough for us to see.

6. Radiation to reproductive organs is especially risky because damage may occur not only to the person but also to genetic material that may be passed on to offspring as a mutation or defect.

7. X-rays cannot pass through lead, which is completely radiopaque, just as light cannot go through the wall of a house.

Answers to Applications

1. This refers to the number of waves that pass a given point in 1 second. In the case of a frequency of 6 Hz a total of 6 waves go by in 1 second.

2. 300 million waves would pass by in 1 second with a frequency of 300 MHz and a wave length of 1 m.

3. 10^{-8} meters. Remember the simple equation: velocity equals frequency times wavelength. Therefore, to calculate wavelength, divide the velocity by the frequency. That is, $3 \times 10^8 \div 3 \times 10^{16}$. That is the same as $1/10^8$, or 10^8.

4. 7.5×10^{14}. If velocity equals frequency times wavelength, then frequency must equal velocity (3×10^8) divided by wavelength (4×10^{-7}).

5. During the de-excitation process the electron returns to its normal shell and emits the higher energy it acquired while being pushed out of it. The energy it emits is in the form of a light photon.

6. You must move 3 m, based on the inverse square law, which states that the intensity of the light diminishes by a factor of the square of the distance from its source. If the light intensity is 1 at 1 m, then it is 1/4 at 2 m and 1/9 at 3 m.

Electrodynamics

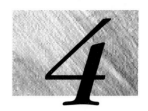

Self-Assessment Pretest

Use this pretest to assess your knowledge of the material in this module before you begin to work through the following exercises. Circle the one answer for each of the following questions. The answers are at the end of this module.

1. What is the term that refers to the principles of nonmoving electric charges?
   a. Electromagnetism
   b. Electrodynamics
   c. Electrostatics

2. Lightning is made of:
   a. Photons
   b. Electrons
   c. Charged protons
   d. Pure energy

3. An electric field extends straight out from an object that is:
   a. Positively charged
   b. Negatively charged
   c. Neutral

4. Electric potential in an electric circuit can be measured by:
   a. An ammeter
   b. A voltmeter
   c. An ohmmeter

5. Electric current is the movement of:
   a. Atoms
   b. Electrons
   c. Alpha particles
   d. Pure energy

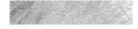

6. Elements or substances that have all electrons bound within the molecules are used as
   a. Conductors
   b. Resistors
   c. Fuses
   d. Insulators

7. The number of electrons flowing past a given point is measured by:
   a. An ammeter
   b. A voltmeter
   c. An ohmmeter

8. Direct current is most commonly used in
   a. Large appliances
   b. Household lighting
   c. Flashlights

9. In comparing a 100-watt light bulb with a 200-watt light bulb, the 200-watt light has half the:
   a. Resistance
   b. Conductivity
   c. Volts
   d. Amperes

10. An electric ground is:
    a. A fuse
    b. A resistor
    c. A protective device
    d. All of the above

Key Terms

Before continuing, be sure you can define the following key terms.

Alternating current: the type of current in which electrons alternate direction of flow as the electric potential switches back and forth.

Alternator: the generator that creates alternating current.

Ammeter: an instrument that measures the electric current in a circuit in amperes; symbolized in standard electric circuit schematics by a circle with an A in it.

Ampere: the SI unit (abbreviated as A) for electrons per second, or how many electrons are flowing past a particular point in the current in 1 second; 1 A equals 1 coulomb flowing by in 1 second.

Circuit breaker: a device that acts in the same manner as a fuse. If the current flowing through it rises above a certain level, the circuit breaker flips its internal switch to open the circuit and stop the electric flow.

Conductor: a metal or other substance with electrons that are free to produce a current.

Contact: one of three forms on electrification of an object; occurs by touching the object so that the charge transfers it.

Coulomb: the SI unit (abbreviated as C) equal to the electric charge of 6.25×10^{18} electrons. This is a negative number for a negative charge; a positive charge of 1 C is equal to the same number of protons.

Coulomb's law: the principle that electrostatic force increases directly as the product of the two charges increases. The force decreases in an inverse relation with the square of the distance between the two objects.

Direct current: the type of current that flows in only one direction; the current produced by batteries.

Electric circuit: the pathway of an electric current.

Electric current: the flow of electrons from the negative charge to the positive charge.

Electric field: the aura in space around a charged object, similar to the gravitational field that exists around a mass. A field is *not* radiation of energy, such as gamma rays or other electromagnetic radiation. Rather, it is like an extension of the charge of the object itself out into the space around it.

Electric ground: a third wire that, in addition to the two wires that conduct the current to and from the circuitry, connects with the wall socket and is wired to a ground source in the building, such as plumbing pipes.

Electric potential: potential energy. In a battery, for example, many electrons are crowded together at the negative battery terminal. The potential is the difference between the charge at the negative end and the charge at the positive end.

Electric power: similar to mechanical power; the rate of doing work.

Electrification: the condition of an object that has gained a charge through friction, contact, or induction.

Electrodynamics: the principles of electric charges in motion.

Electrostatic force: the force of attraction or repulsion between charged objects. The amount of force present depends on the amount of electric charge in each object and the distance between them.

Electrostatics: the principles of nonmoving electric charges.

Friction: one of three forms of electrification of an object; occurs by rubbing electrons off one object and depositing them on another.

Fuse: a section of special wire, usually encased in glass, that quickly melts if the current flowing through it rises too high.

Ground: something that is able to absorb electric charges.

Induction: one of three forms of electrification of an object; occurs when one charged object attracts the opposite charges in another object and thereby electrifies that area of the other object.

Insulator: a substance that does not conduct electric current because its electrons are bound within the molecules and cannot freely move.

Ion: the result of electrons moving in or out of their electron shells; an ion has a positive or negative charge.

Joule: the SI unit for energy, abbreviated as J; the ability to do work.

Measuring device: an instrument used to measure electric properties in a system or circuit.

Ohm: the SI unit for resistance, symbolized by the Greek letter omega (Ω).

Ohmmeter: an instrument that measures the resistance of a resistor or a section of circuit between its two probes; symbolized in standard electric circuit schematics by a circle with an O in it.

Ohm's law: the principle that potential difference equals the current flow times resistance.

Open circuit: a break in a circuit that stops the flow of electrons.

Protective device: an object, such as a circuit breaker, that protects an electric circuit and the human beings around it if something goes wrong.

Resistance: the ability of an element in a circuit to resist the flow of electricity by reducing or impeding it.

Schematic: a diagram of an electric circuit.

Short circuit: an unintended pathway that allows the current to pass directly across the electric potential instead of through an element that uses the power.

Static: nonmoving, such as an electric charge at rest; differentiates an electrostatic charge from a flowing electric current.

Volts: the unit of measurement (abbreviated as V) for electric potential; the difference in electric charge between two points.

Voltmeter: an instrument that measures the electric potential across the two points touched by its probes; symbolized in standard electric circuit schematics by a circle with a V in it.

Watt: the SI unit for electric power, abbreviated as W.

Topical Outline

The following material is covered in this module.

I. Electrostatics involves the principles of nonmoving electric charges.
   A. Coulomb's law states that electrostatic force increases directly as the product of the two charges increases. The force decreases in an inverse relation with the square of the distance between the two objects.
   B. Electric charge refers to the positive, negative, or neutral state of an object.
   C. Electric field is the aura in space around a charged object. A field is *not* radiation of energy, such as gamma rays or other electromagnetic radiation. Rather, it is like an extension of the charge of the object itself out into the space around it.
   D. Electrification of an object occurs when it gains a charge through friction, contact, or induction.

II. Electrodynamics is the term for the principles of electric charges in motion.
   A. Electric current is the flow of electrons from the negative charge to the positive charge.
      1. Alternating current is the type of current in which electrons alternate direction of flow as the electric potential switches back and forth.
      2. Direct current is the type of current that flows in only one direction. It is the current produced by batteries.
   B. Potential refers to potential energy. Electric potential is the difference between the charge at the negative end and the charge at the positive end.
   C. Resistance is the ability of an element in a circuit to resist the flow of electricity by reducing or impeding it.
   D. Conductors are metals and other substances with electrons that are free to produce a current.
   E. Circuits are the pathways of an electric current.

III. Basic electric devices are instruments that measure or protect an electric system.
   A. Measuring devices measure electric properties in a system or circuit.
   B. Protective devices safeguard an electric circuit and the human beings around it if something goes wrong.

Review

1. As illustrated by the figure below, electrons can be bumped into or out of _electron shells_ in atoms, creating positively or negatively charged _ion_ .

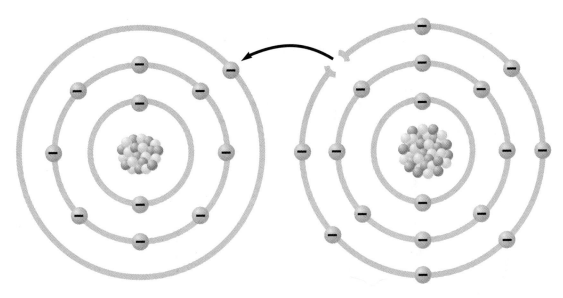

MOVEMENT OF ELECTRONS AFFECTS CHANGE OF PARTICLES

2. Lightning is another example of _stactic_ electricity. Clouds in a storm may lose or gain electrons as the wind, air molecules, and water molecules interact. _Electron_ from a negatively charged cloud may jump to a _postive_ charged cloud or to the _neutral_ earth.

3. A voltmeter, symbolized in standard electric circuit _Schematic_ by a circle with a _V_ in it, measures the electric potential across the two points touched by its probes. In the illustration below, the voltmeter measures the _Voltage_ of the battery in the circuit. A V is equal to the amount of _work_ that can be done per unit charge.

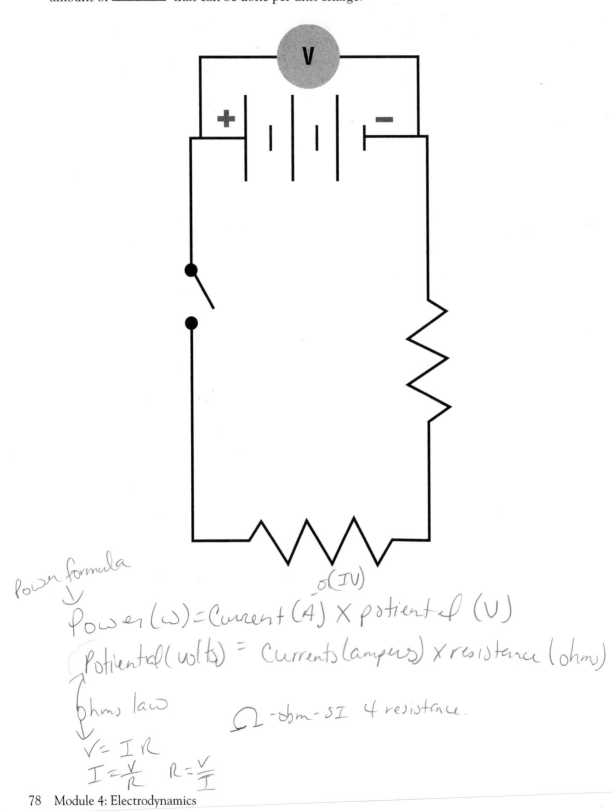

Power formula ↓

Power (W) = Current (A) X potiential (U) ₒ(IU)

Potiential (volts) = Currents (ampers) x resistance (ohms)

Ohms law

Ω -ohm-SI 4 resistance.

V = IR
I = V/R   R = V/I

4. An ammeter, symbolized in standard electric circuit schematics by a circle with an ___*A*___ in it, measures the ___current___ in a circuit in amperes (A). In the illustration below, the ammeter measures the current in the loop created with the battery and the two ___resistor___. Note that the switch has to be closed for the ___curcuit___ to be complete in order for the current to run. If the switch had been open, the ammeter would register ___0___ current. An A is the SI unit for the flow of electrons per second.

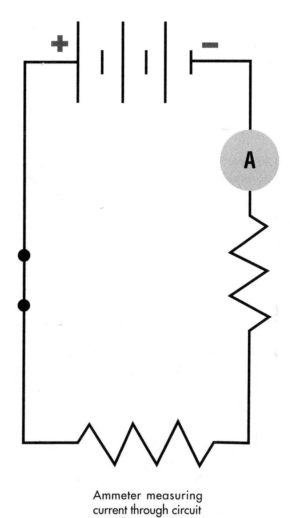

Ammeter measuring
current through circuit

5. An ohmmeter, symbolized in standard electric _Circuit_ schematics by a circle with an O in it, measures the _resistance_ of a resistor or a section of circuit between its two probes. In the illustration below, the ohmmeter measures the resistance of one _resistor_ in the circuit.

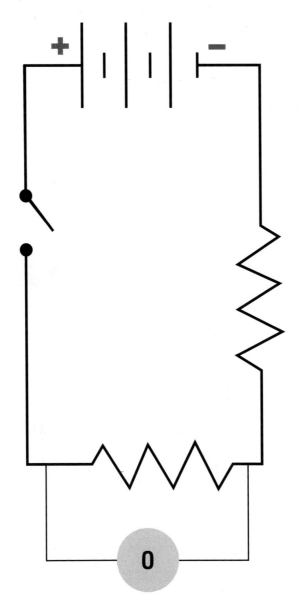

6. Electric power is the same as mechanical power: the ___rate___ of doing work. Thus we talk about how much ___power___ an electric appliance uses. The SI unit for electric power is the ___W___; 1 watt is the rate of 1 ___A___ of current across a potential of 1 volt.

7. As illustrated by the figure below, when you walk across a wool rug, ___electrons___ are rubbed from the wool fibers onto your shoes. As you attract more electrons, your whole body gains a ___negative___ charge. The extra electrons on your body are ___repelled___ from each other and seek to escape from you. When you reach out to a metal doorknob or another person, either of which has a charge that is ___neutral___ compared to you, the extra electrons jump from your fingers to escape. You feel this as a shock of ___static___ electricity.

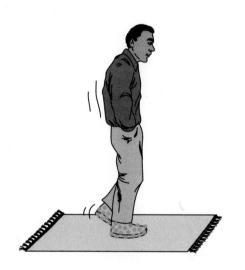

PICKING UP AN
ELECTROSTATIC CHARGE

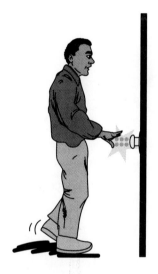

LOSING THE CHARGE
IN A SPARK!

8. The figure below represents an electric field force of attraction and _repulsion_. Two objects with the same _charge_ repel each other. The fields of two _positive_ charges push each other away. The fields of two negative charges _pull_ away from each other. Two objects with _opposite_ charges attract each other. The field of the positive one pushes in the same direction as the pull of the _negative_ one. The forces in these two fields add up because they are in the same direction.

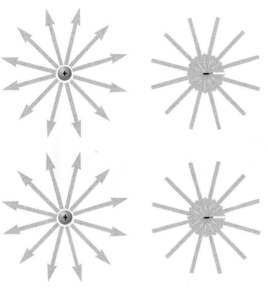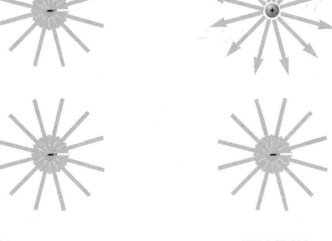

REPULSION   ATTRACTION

9. Electrostatic force is the _electrication_ of objects when they gain a charge. An object can be electrified in three ways: _friction_, which rubs electrons off one object and deposits them on another; _contact_, such as when a charged fingertip touches a doorknob and the charge moves to the metal; and _induction_, when one charged object attracts the opposite charges in another object and thereby electrifies that area of the other object.

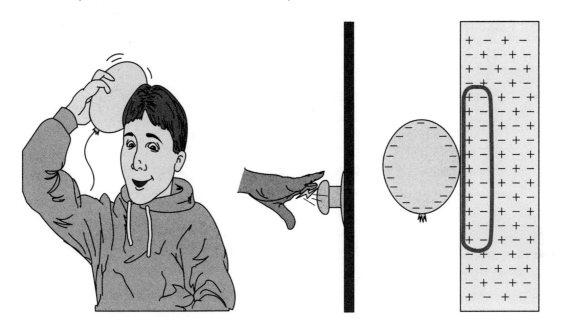

10. The figure below represents the atoms in most nonmetallic elements. These elements do not _conduct_ electric current, however. In the atoms of these elements the _electrons_ are generally bound within the molecules and cannot freely move to produce a current, even when attracted by a potential difference. These substances are called _insulators_.

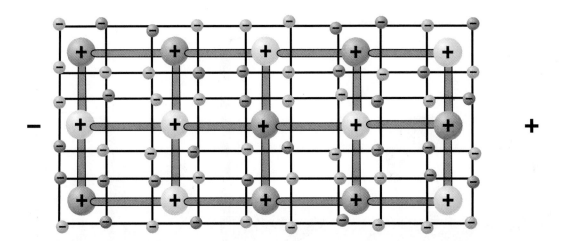

Electrons Not Free To Move
Even When Potential Applied

11. There are two types of electric current, _direct_ and alternating. As shown in the illustration below, in alternating current the _electrons_ alternate direction of flow as the electric _potential_ switches back and forth.

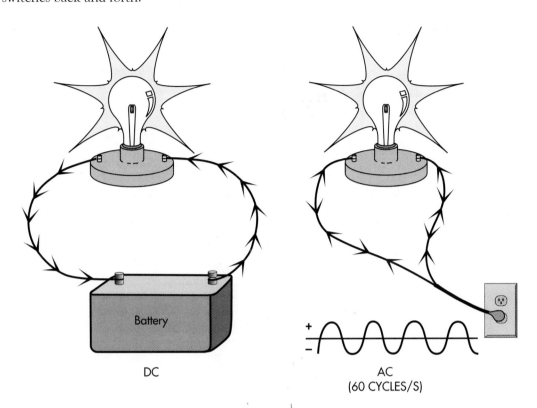

DC

AC
(60 CYCLES/S)

12. Protective electric devices safeguard the _circuit,_ and the human beings around it, if something goes wrong. Wires may break or cross, creating a _short circuit_ that can produce dangerously high currents and sparks or fire. Dangerous electric shocks are also possible with damaged equipment, especially with high- _voltage_ equipment such as x-ray machines.

13. As illustrated by the earlier figure, batteries always have a _negative_ terminal and a _positive_ terminal, and the current always flows out of one terminal and into the other. This current always moves _directly_ from one side of the _potential_ to the other.

14. Inside the battery shown below, the negative _ions_ cannot reach the positive zinc ions to which they are _attracted_, but they can flow out the negative terminal of the battery and through a conductor to reach the positive terminal. This is an example of a _direct_ current.

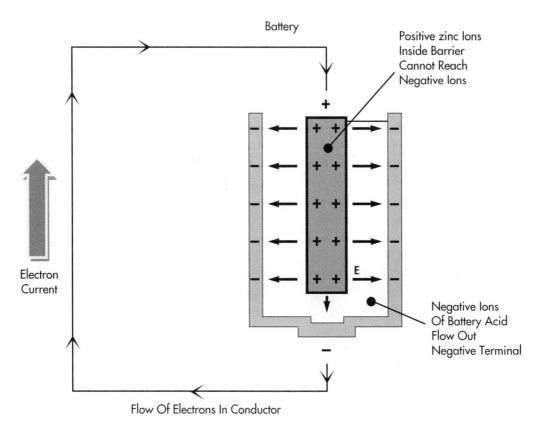

Battery

Positive zinc Ions
Inside Barrier
Cannot Reach
Negative Ions

+

E

Electron
Current

Negative Ions
Of Battery Acid
Flow Out
Negative Terminal

−

Flow Of Electrons In Conductor

15. If an electrical current is broken by opening a circuit, such as by turning a switch off, then the _electron_ flow stops. This is sometimes called an _open_ circuit. If an unintended pathway occurs that allows the current to pass directly across the electric potential instead of through an element that uses the power, then a _short_ circuit occurs.

16. A circuit breaker acts in the same manner as a _fuse_. If the current flowing through it rises above a certain level, the _circuit_ breaker flips its internal switch to open the circuit and stop the _electric_ flow.

Learning Quiz

The following material is similar to the interactive exercises found in the CD-ROM version of this module operated in the "student mode." These questions will allow you to review the concepts presented in this module and will help you to gain a more complete understanding of the material.

1. If the electric charge of a wall is neutral, why will a balloon that has picked up extra electrons stick to it?

2. If the electrons in lightning moved at the speed of light, they would hit the ground before your eyes ever saw them. What is happening that allows you to see the lightning?

3. How is the change in intensity of light at a distance from the source similar to the change in electrostatic force?

4. Lightning is a form of static electricity and is measured in terms of electric potential. How does the electric potential of lightning change?

5. What are the two measures of the strength of an electric current?

6. What type of energy in a battery is used to create electric energy?

7. Consider that a resistor of 100 Ω is placed near the beginning of an electrical circuit, and a second resistor with half the Ω is placed 2 m away on the same circuit. Will the current change after it passes the second resistor, and is the current before the first resistor different from the current after the first resistor?

8. Why does the current in an electric circuit increase when there is a short circuit?

Applications

1. In a 100 A electric service, how many C will flow by in 1 second?

2. If two charged objects are moved three times as far apart, what will be the change in force?

3. Here is a two-part question based on Coulomb's law. Assuming two objects stay the same distance apart, if one object has a charge of 2 C and the other object has a charge of 6 C, what is the total force? If the first object then doubles to 4 C while the second object remains at 6 C what is the total force?

4. What two conditions must be met for an electric current to exist?

5. If the potential of a household circuit is 110 V, how many A are flowing through the circuit to power a 60 W light bulb?

6. If you know that the voltage in your house is 110 V and your handy ammeter reads 0.91 A in a particular circuit, how many W is the bulb on the electric circuit?

7. What is the resistance in Ω of a light bulb if the voltage is 110 V and the amperage is 0.91 A?

8. If the resistor in an electric circuit is changed so the Ω are cut in half, what will happen to the A?

Posttest

Circle the best answer for each of the following questions. Your instructor has the correct answers.

1. Electrostatics involves the principles of:
   a. All electric charges
   b. Nonmoving electric charges
   c. Moving electric charges

2. Which of the following best describes an electric charge?
   a. A photon
   b. A particle
   c. A property of a particle

3. Protons in the nucleus of an atom:
   a. Attract each other
   b. Repel each other
   c. Are neutral

4. What is created when electrons are bumped into or out of electron shells?
   a. Ions
   b. Isotopes
   c. Isotones
   d. Isobars

5. When the earth is struck by lightning, the ground:
   a. Becomes positively charged
   b. Becomes negatively charged
   c. Stays neutral

6. The SI unit that is equal to 6.25×10^{18} electrons or protons is called:
   a. Ampere
   b. Coulomb
   c. Watt

7. An electric field extends straight toward an object from all directions that is:
   a. Positively charged
   b. Negatively charged
   c. Neutral

8. The force of attraction or repulsion between charged objects is called:
   a. Electrodynamics
   b. Electrostatic field
   c. Electrostatic force
   d. Electromagnetic force

9. When electrons rub off one object and are deposited on another, this is said to be electrification by:
   a. Contact
   b. Induction
   c. Friction

10. What is the process by which one charged object attracts the opposite charges in another object and thereby electrifies that area of the other object?
    a. Contact
    b. Induction
    c. Friction
    d. Generation

11. What is the term for the principles of electric charges in motion?
    a. Electrodynamics
    b. Electrostatics
    c. Electrification

12. Potential energy is:
    a. Electric current
    b. The ability to transmit current
    c. The ability to do work

13. The difference in electric charge between two points is measured in:
    a. Amperes
    b. Ohms
    c. Volts
    d. Watts

14. A "liquid"-like free flow of electrons in metal is characteristic of:
    a. Insulators
    b. Resistors
    c. Conductors
    d. All elements

15. Atoms in which electrons are generally bound within the molecules and cannot freely move are characteristically found in:
    a. Insulators
    b. Resistors
    c. Conductors
    d. All nonmetallic substances

16. The SI unit for electrons per second is:
    a. Amperes
    b. Ohms *resistan*
    c. Volts
    d. Watts
    e. Coulombs

17. What type of current do batteries produce?
    a. Alternating
    b. Direct
    c. Stored voltage

18. The standard electricity that flows into your house is a current that alternates in direction at:
    a. 200 cycles per second
    b. 40 cycles per second
    c. 60 cycles per second
    d. 80 cycles per second

19. What is the SI unit for electric power?
    a. Amperes
    b. Ohms
    c. Volts
    d. Watts
    e. Coulombs

20. Power in W equals A times:
    a. Coulombs
    b. Ohms
    c. Volts

21. What is the pathway of an electric current called?
    a. Open circuit
    b. Electric circuit
    c. Conductor
    d. Schematic

22. An open circuit refers to:
    a. The pathway for electric current
    b. Stopping the flow of electrons
    c. Allowing the flow of electrons

23. What is a device called that impedes or reduces the flow of electricity?
    a. Circuit breaker
    b. Fuse
    c. Resistor
    d. Insulator

24. As resistance increases, current in an electric circuit:
    a. Decreases
    b. Increases
    c. Does not change

25. What is the SI unit for resistance called?
    a. Ampere
    b. Ohm
    c. Volt
    d. Watt
    e. Coulomb

26. In comparing 200- and 100-watt light bulbs, the 200-watt bulb has:
    a. Twice the resistance
    b. Half the resistance
    c. The same resistance

27. Circuits in complex equipment may have:
    a. Different voltages
    b. Varying resistances
    c. Different currents
    d. All of the above
    e. None of the above

28. What is the device called that measures the amount of electric current flowing through a circuit at a particular point?
    a. Ammeter
    b. Ohmmeter
    c. Voltmeter

29. Which of the following is considered a protective device?
    a. A fuse
    b. A circuit breaker
    c. A ground
    d. All of the above

30. The ground wire in electric equipment is connected to the:
    a. Equipment circuit
    b. Equipment housing
    c. Negative terminal
    d. Positive terminal

Answer Key

Answers to Pretest

1. c

2. b

3. a

4. b

5. b

6. d

7. a

8. c

9. a

10. c

Answers to Review

1. Electron shells, ions

2. Static, Electrons, positively, neutral

3. Schematics, V, potential (or voltage), work

4. A, electric current, resistors, circuit, zero

5. Circuit, resistance, resistor

6. Rate, power, W, A

7. Electrons, negative, repelled, neutral, static

8. Repulsion, charge, positive, pull, opposite, negative

9. Electrification, friction, contact, induction

10. Conduct, electrons, insulators

11. Direct, electrons, potential

12. Circuit, short circuit, voltage

13. Negative, positive, potential

14. Ions, attracted, direct

15. Electron (or electric), open, short

16. Fuse, circuit, electric (or electron)

Answers to Learning Quiz

1. It seems odd at first to think that an object with a neutral charge, like the wall in this example, can still have charges moving about within it. Remember, however, that neutrality is just a balance of positive and negative charges, just as gray is a balanced mix of white and black. If something pulled on all the white parts of a gray picture, for example, the white could separate out and pull to one side, leaving the black on the other side. That's what happens with the wall: the positive charges are pulled to the surface near the balloon, even though the wall as a whole remains neutral.

2. Although an electric field moves at the speed of light, electrons themselves take more time to get where they are going, whether through a wire to a light bulb or through the air in a lightning bolt. That is why you can actually see the bolt of lightning move across the sky. If the electrons moved at the speed of light, they would be at the other end long before you even had time to realize they had started!

3. The inverse square law of light means that as you get farther from a light source, the intensity of the light diminishes according to the square of the distance between you and the source. The same inverse relationship applies to electrostatic force.

4. Just before the bolt of lightning strikes, there may be an electric potential of hundreds of millions of V between the cloud and the earth. Thus the lightning has a great deal of energy, but it is not sustained energy that produces an electric current; it is only but a momentary flash, after which there is no longer any electric potential.

5. The two measures of the strength of an electric current are V and A. A low-voltage, high-amperage current has many moving electrons, but they are not as powerful because the electric potential is lower. A low-amperage, high-voltage current has fewer moving electrons, but they are more powerful because the electric potential is higher.

6. Batteries convert chemical energy to electric energy. Energy is never created or destroyed—it can only be converted from one form to another.

7. The answer to both questions is no. The *whole* circuit is affected by resistance at any one point. If only a small amount of current can get by the first resistor, then only the same amount will flow by the second resistor. In addition, the current before the resistor is also restricted. This is similar to the flow of water in a pipe. If a large pipe is reduced to a small pipe, the flow of water in both is restricted. When the small pipe is enlarged, the flow of water is still only equal to the flow in the small pipe. Even in the section of pipe *before* the thin section, the flow is reduced to the same amount. It is like a large crowd funneling out one doorway of a room—the whole crowd can move at the rate of only one person at a time.

8. There is an inverse relation between resistance and current: as one factor goes up, the other goes down. The less resistance, the more current; the more resistance, the less current. In a short circuit the resistance is bypassed so there is almost no resistance, and thus the current can be extremely large.

Answers to Applications

1. 100 coulombs, since 1 ampere equals 1 coulomb flowing by in 1 second.

2. Based on Coulomb's law the force will follow the inverse square. In this case the inverse square of 3 is $\frac{1}{9}$.

3. The answers here are very simple. The total force of two objects is the product of the two objects. In this case $2 \times 6 = 12$ as total force. Secondly, $4 \times 6 = 24$.

4. First, there must be an electric potential difference between two charges, and second, there must be a pathway for electrons to travel between the two charges.

5. The answer is 0.55 amperes since power in watts equals current in amperes times the potential in volts. The equation to find amperes is watts (60) divided by volts (110).

6. The answer is 100 watts, or 0.91 amperes $\times$ 110 volts.

7. The answer is 120.9 ohms, or 110 volts divided by 0.91 amperes.

8. The amperes will double. Since there is now half the resistance, twice the current will be able to flow.

Electromagnetism

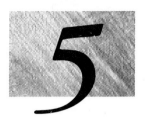

Self-Assessment Pretest

Use this pretest to assess your knowledge of the material in this module before you begin to work through the following exercises. Circle the best answer for each of the following questions. The answers to pretest questions are at the end of this module.

1. An electric field exists around any charged particle. When the charged particles move, what is produced?
   a. A magnetic field
   b. An alternating current
   c. A direct current

2. To which of the following can the inverse square law be applied?
   a. Electromagnetic radiation
   b. Magnetic fields
   c. Electric fields
   d. All of the above

3. Iron is ferromagnetic and rubber nonmagnetic. The element cobalt is:
   a. Ferromagnetic
   b. Nonmagnetic
   c. Paramagnetic

4. Magnetic domains are:
   a. Magnetic fields
   b. Aligned atoms that produce a magnetic field
   c. Natural magnetic material

5. A permanent magnet placed in the middle of a coil is called:
   a. An electromagnet
   b. A solenoid
   c. An armature
   d. A rotor

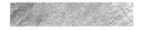

6. Moving a wire through a magnetic field induces:
   a. A current
   b. A magnetic field
   c. Resistance

7. In electromagnetic induction, current can be increased by increasing:
   a. The strength of the magnet
   b. The speed of motion of the coil
   c. The number of coils
   d. All of the above
   e. None of the above

8. What is the process called when the current in one coil produces a current in another coil?
   a. Self-induction
   b. Auto-induction
   c. Mutual induction

9. Slip rings and brushes in an electric generator are used to produce:
   a. Alternating current
   b. Direct current
   c. Both of the above
   d. Neither of the above

10. What type of electric motor uses electromagnets rather than fixed magnets?
    a. An alternating-current motor
    b. A direct-current motor
    c. An induction motor

Key Terms

Before continuing, be sure you can define the following key terms.

Alternating-current motor: a motor that works by the current alternating its direction, which causes the magnetic field around the coils to alternate polarity. This moving polarity causes the coils in the motor to turn.

Armature: a coil of wire that rotates inside a magnetic field to produce an electric current. The more turns of wire in the coil, the higher the voltage induced in the wire.

Artificial permanent magnet: a magnet that is manufactured, in which the alignment of the atoms is induced by a process that turns an object into a magnet.

Autotransformer: a transformer in which the wire is wound only once around the magnetic core. This one winding is used as both the primary and secondary coils. The outside wires are attached at different points along the coil, and the induced voltage varies depending on where the connections are made.

Closed-core transformer: a transformer in which the material on the top and bottom of the two coil cores helps to contain and direct the magnetic force lines.

Core: the ferromagnetic material around which the coils are wrapped. This material becomes magnetic along with the coils, which increases and focuses the overall magnetic field within a transformer.

Dipole: a magnetic field that is created by a single electron.

Direct-current motor: a motor in which a commutator ring with rotating contacts or brushes reverses the current's direction in the coils as they move in and out of the magnetic field of the permanent magnets. This ensures that the motor keeps turning in one direction.

Electric field: an alteration of the space around a charge.

Electric generator: a generator that produces an electric current by rotating loops of wire through a fixed magnetic field.

Electric motor: a motor in which current is supplied to create a magnetic field around the coils, which are moved by the magnetic field of the stronger permanent magnets surrounding the coil. This motion makes the motor turn.

Electromagnet: an object that creates a temporary magnetic field through the flow of electricity. It has many applications in electric equipment.

Electromagnetic induction: a current that is induced to flow in a wire by moving the wire through a magnetic field or by moving a magnetic field through the wire.

Electromagnetism: the movement of electrons in an electric current, which creates a magnetic field.

Ferromagnetic material: a substance, such as iron, that is attracted to a magnet.

Induction: the process by which iron atoms become aligned and thus turn an object into a magnet. Magnetism is said to be induced in such a situation.

Induction motor: a very powerful motor that can be controlled to rotate at any speed because the strength of the magnetic fields can be controlled, as can the timing of the series of outside electromagnetic fields. The magnetic field around the coils in the center is created by a series of electromagnets rather than fixed magnets.

Inverse square law: the principle that a magnetic field is proportional to the product of the magnetic force of each pole divided by the square of the distance between the poles.

Lenz's law: the principle that an induced current flows in the opposite direction of the magnetic field that induced it.

Magnetic domain: a property of magnets that occurs when many atoms align to produce a larger magnetic field.

Magnetic field: the area around moving charged particles. It exerts a magnetic force on certain kinds of particles within the field.

Mutual induction: the phenomenon in which one current induces another current.

Natural magnet: a permanent magnet, known as a lodestone, that is a rock with a natural magnetic force acquired from the earth's magnetic field. A lodestone remains magnetic unless something happens to change its arrangement of electrons.

Nonmagnetic material: a substance in which the magnetic forces caused by the spin of some electrons is neutralized by the spin of other electrons.

Paramagnetic material: a substance that has a very weak attraction to magnetic fields.

Polarity: a term referring to the north and south poles of a magnetic field.

Principles of magnetic fields: three laws of magnetic fields, which are: (1) unlike magnetic poles attract and like magnetic poles repel; (2) all magnets and all magnetic fields have both a north and south pole; (3) magnetic fields follow the inverse square law.

Self-induction: the process that occurs in a single coil of wire when an alternating current flows through it. The flow of electrons in one direction produces a magnetic field.

Shell transformer: the most commonly used transformer; it "traps" the magnetic forces more efficiently in order to induce the strongest possible current in the secondary coil.

Solenoid: a device that is made by positioning a permanent magnet core in the middle of the coils, thereby increasing the strength of an electromagnet's magnetic field.

Tesla: the SI unit (abbreviated as T) used to measure the strength of a magnetic field.

Transformer: a device that changes the electric potential to a higher or lower voltage and also raises or lowers the current. Transformers are used for this purpose in x-ray equipment circuitry.

Transformer law: the principle that there is a direct proportion between the ratio of wire turns and the ratio of voltage.

Topical Outline

The following material is covered in this module.

I. Magnetism is closely related to electric force. Each of these forces is part of the phenomenon called electromagnetism. When charged particles move, a magnetic field is produced around them.
   A. Magnets are created from materials in which the atoms line up in a set way so that all the free electrons spin in the same direction.
   B. A dipole is the magnetic field created by a single electron.
   C. A magnetic domains is created when many atoms align to produce a larger magnetic field.
   D. Induction is the process of aligning the atoms and turning an object into a magnet.
   E. Magnetic fields are similar to electrostatic fields in that opposite poles attract and like poles repel.
   F. The inverse square law applies to magnetism as it does electromagnetic radiation.

II. The principles of electromagnetism explain how x-rays are produced and how radiographic equipment works.
   A. Electromagnets are temporary magnetic fields created by the flow of electricity. They have many applications in electric equipment.
   B. The strength of an electromagnetic field can be increased in a number of ways: by increasing the strength of the magnet, the number of coils, or the speed of motion of the coil through the magnetic field.
   C. Electromagnetic induction is the process of creating a current by moving a wire through a magnetic field or by moving a magnetic field through a coil of wire.
   D. Electromagnetic fields do not extend outward in a straight line, but curve back around toward the magnet's other pole.

III. Electric equipment is based on the principles of electromagnetism and induction.
   A. Electric generators produce an electric current by rotating loops of wire through a fixed magnetic field.
   B. Electric motors supply a current that creates a magnetic field around the coils, which are moved by the magnetic field of the stronger permanent magnets surrounding the coil. This motion makes the motor turn.
   C. Coils, or armatures, are loops of wires that rotate inside a magnetic field. The more turns of wire in the coil, the higher the voltage induced in the wire.
   D. Transformers operate on the principles of electromagnetic induction. When an alternating current flows through the primary coil, the collapsing and expanding magnetic field that is created will induce a current in the secondary coil.

Review

1. As shown in the figure below, an electric field exists around any _charged particle_ or object. A field is an alteration of the space around that charge. This field exerts an _electric force_ on any particle within the field. When charged particles move, a _magnetic field_ is produced around them.

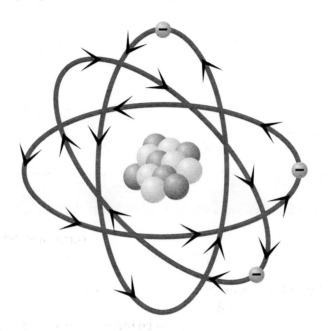

Every Moving
Charge Produces
A Magnetic Field

2. Because the electrons in most substances spin in all different directions, the magnetic fields are canceled out, or made _neutral_, in most objects. In magnetized iron the atoms line up in a set way so that all the free _electrons_ spin in the same direction. Then all those tiny magnetic fields with millions of individual electrons add up to make one bigger _magnetic field_

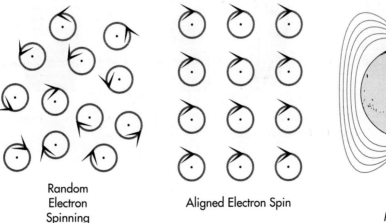

Random
Electron
Spinning

Aligned Electron Spin

Earth's
Magnetic
Field

3. As illustrated by the figure below, unlike magnetic poles _attract_ and like magnetic poles _repel_ . The north pole of a magnet attracts the _South_ pole of another magnet but repels its north pole. This applies also to the whole _magnetic field_ , not just the poles.

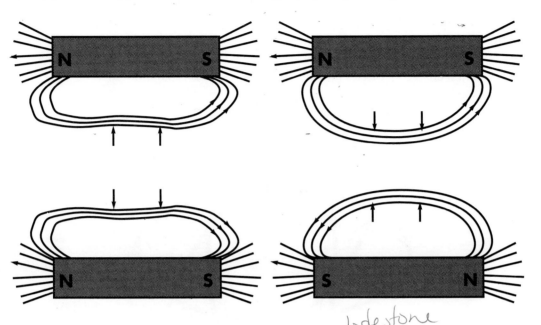

4. Natural magnets are found on the earth and are often called _lodestone_ . A second type of magnet is manufactured and is called an _Artificial permanent magnet_ . Most of the magnets we see are created this way. A third type is the electromagnet, which creates a _temporary_ magnetic field through the flow of electricity.

TYPES OF MAGNETS

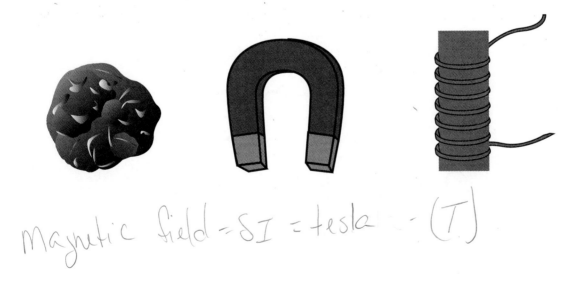

Magnetic field = SI = tesla - (T)

5. The direction of magnetic field lines can be determined by using what is called the _right hand rule_. As shown in the figure below, if the thumb of your right hand points in the direction of the current flowing through a wire, then the direction of the magnetic field circles the wire in the _same_ direction as the fingers.

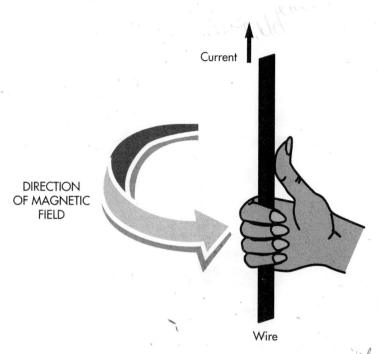

Current

DIRECTION
OF MAGNETIC
FIELD

Wire

6. An electromagnet can be created by a current that is flowing through a _wire coil_. As illustrated by the figure below, positioning a _permanent magnet_ in the middle of the coils increases the strength of the electromagnet's magnetic field. This is called a _solenoid_.

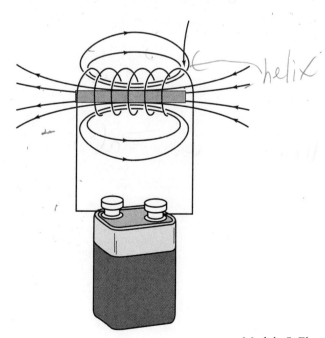

helix

7. Which end of a magnetic field is the north pole and which is the south pole is referred to as
polarity . As the current _alternates_, what was first the north pole now becomes the south, then the north again, and so on, making a kind of _pulsing_ in and out of the field.

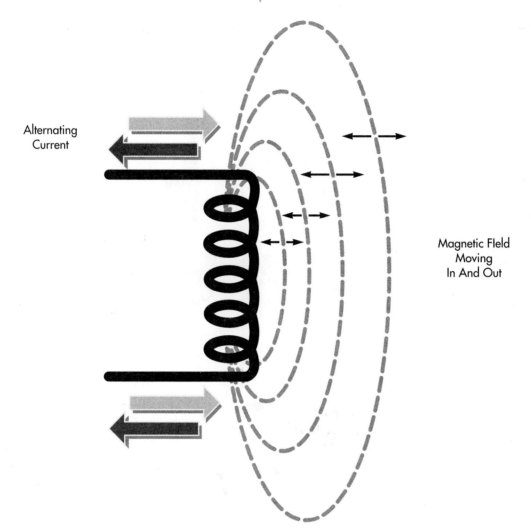

Alternating
Current

Magnetic Field
Moving
In And Out

8. If you put another coil of wire next to one that is generating a pulsing magnetic field, a current is induced in the _2nd coil_ because there is relative _motion_ between it and the moving magnetic field created by the first coil. The first coil, which generates the _magnetic_ field, is called the primary coil. The second coil, in which a _current_ is induced by the magnetic field, is called the secondary coil.

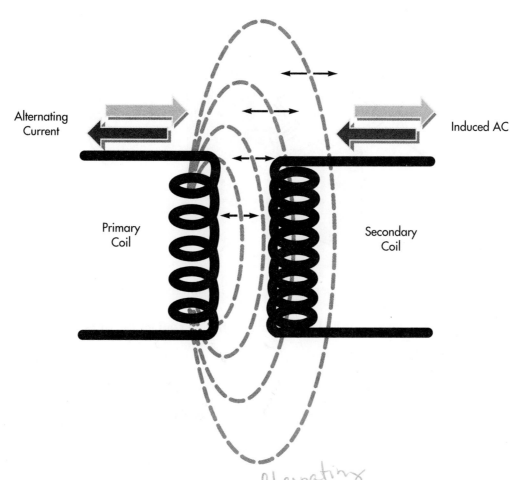

Alternating Current

Induced AC

Primary Coil

Secondary Coil

9. In a secondary coil the induced current is an _alternating_ current because of the continually switching _polarity_ of the magnetic field. This is called _mutual induction_, referring to the process in which one current induces another current.

10. In the figure below, the current generated in the wire of the loop or coil is always an _alternating_ current. If the _generator_ parts are configured so that the current of the wire coil is conducted directly from the generator to an electric circuit, the whole circuit is an _alternating_ current.

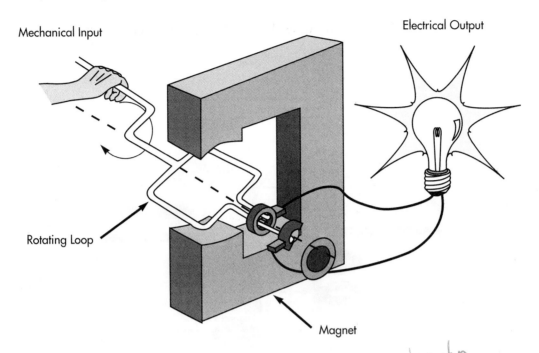

Mechanical Input

Electrical Output

Rotating Loop

Magnet

11. A direct current generator can be constructed by adding slip rings and _brushes_ to the ends of the _coil_ in the generator. The brushes outside the coil contact the wires of the coil in an _alternating_ manner.

12. The purpose of transformers is to change the electric potential, to a higher or lower _voltage_. X-ray production typically requires very _high_ voltage, and thus a transformer is included in the circuitry. Transformers also raise or lower the _current_ and are used for this purpose in x-ray equipment circuitry.

13. In transformers the voltage of the _secondary_ coil depends on the ratio of the number of turns of wiring in the _coil_ . For example, if there are twice as many turns in the secondary coil as there are in the primary coil, then the voltage in the secondary coil is _2X_ that of the primary coil. If there are half as many turns in the secondary coil, the voltage is half that in the primary _coil_ .

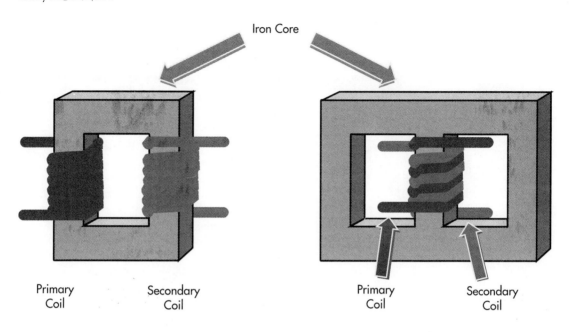

COMMON CONFIGURATIONS OF TRANSFORMERS

14. The two most common types of transformers are the _Closed_ and the _Shell_ . In both, there is a core of magnetic material that strengthens and controls the magnetic field. In the first type, the material on the top and bottom of the two coil cores helps contain and direct the magnetic force lines. The second type "traps" the magnetic forces more efficiently and induces the strongest possible current in the _secondary_ coil.

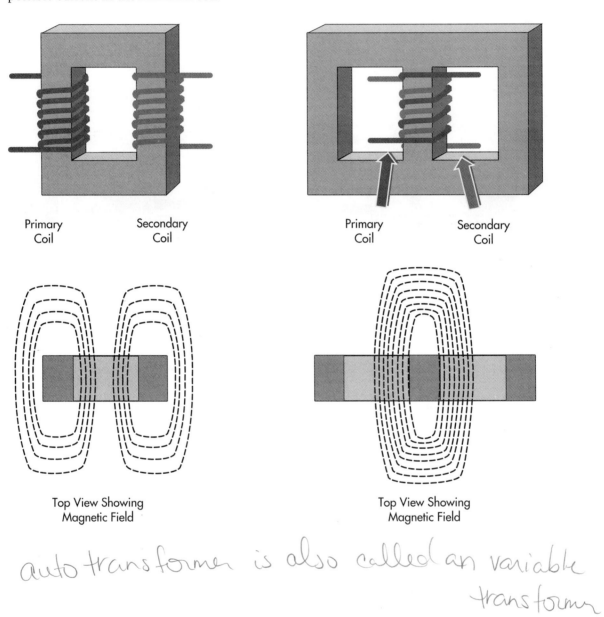

Primary   Secondary
Coil   Coil

Primary   Secondary
Coil   Coil

Top View Showing
Magnetic Field

Top View Showing
Magnetic Field

auto transformer is also called an variable transformer

Learning Quiz

The following material is similar to the interactive exercises found in the CD-ROM version of this module operated in the "student mode." These questions will allow you to review the concepts presented in this module and will help you to gain a more complete understanding of the material.

1. What is the difference between electric fields and magnetic fields in terms of their ability to repel and attract?

2. What effect does a magnet have on the electrons of nonmagnetized iron?

3. Which has a stronger magnetic field, the earth or a refrigerator magnet?

4. What is the difference between induction and electromagnetic induction?

5. What happens to the polarity of an electromagnet that is created by using an alternating current?

6. What is the difference between the direct current produced by a direct current generator and that produced by a battery?

7. What is the core of a closed-core transformer made of, and what is its purpose?

Applications

1. If every electron creates a magnetic field, why is everything not magnetic?

2. Using the inverse square law, determine the change in magnetic intensity. If the intensity is $\frac{1}{10}$ T at 1 mm, what will it be at 3 mm?

3. If the number of coils of wire increases from 75 to 225, what is the increase in magnetic field strength?

4. Imagine one coil has 20 turns of wire, and a magnet is moved in and out of it once every second. Then imagine a second coil with 40 turns of wire and a magnet that is moved in and out three times every second. How much stronger is the current produced by the second coil?

5. If a transformer has a primary-coil voltage of 220 V, and there are 100 turns of wire in the primary coil and 300 turns in the secondary coil, what is the voltage in the secondary coil?

6. If a transformer has a primary coil voltage of 220 V, and there are 100 turns of wire in the primary coil and 50 turns in the secondary coil, what is the voltage in the secondary coil?

7. Why is a compass needle attracted to a wire carrying a current?

Posttest

Circle the best answer for each of the following questions. Your instructor has the correct answers.

1. Every magnet:
   a. Is made out of iron
   b. Has north and south poles
   c. Both of the above
   d. Neither of the above

2. Which of the following is not considered ferromagnetic?
   a. Iron
   b. Lead
   c. Nickel
   d. Cobalt

3. In nonmagnetic materials the magnetic forces caused by the spin of some electrons is neutralized by the spin of:
   a. Neutrons
   b. Protons
   c. Other electrons
   d. All of the above

4. Paramagnetic materials are:
   a. Artificial magnets
   b. Electromagnets
   c. Materials with weak attraction to magnetic fields

5. The magnetic field created by a single electron is called a:
   a. Dipole
   b. Domain
   c. Induced magnetic field
   d. Paramagnet

6. What is naturally occurring magnetic rock called?
   a. Magnesia
   b. Lodestone
   c. Electromagnetic rock

7. What is the process called when iron atoms become aligned and thus turn an object into a magnet?
   a. Magnetism
   b. Generation
   c. Induction
   d. Mutual induction

8. Which of the following will *not* help in the process of turning a ferromagnetic material into a magnet?
   a. Placing it in a magnetic field
   b. Tapping it
   c. Rubbing it against a magnet
   d. Heating it

9. Magnetic field lines:
   a. Radiate out from the point of charge
   b. Radiate into the point of charge
   c. Always stretch from one pole to the other
   d. None of the above

10. What happens as the poles of a magnet are spread farther apart?
    a. The magnet gets stronger
    b. The magnet gets weaker
    c. There is no change in the magnetic force
    d. The magnetic field lines get shorter

11. According to the inverse square law, the strength of a magnetic field is proportional to the product of the magnetic force of each pole divided by the square of the distance between:
    a. Field lines
    b. Fields
    c. Magnets
    d. Poles

12. Which of the following is not considered one of the three basic types of magnets?
    a. Permanent magnets
    b. Natural magnets
    c. Artificial permanent magnets
    d. Electromagnets

13. The term "moving charge" refers to the movement of:
    a. Protons
    b. Current
    c. Electrons
    d. Magnets

14. Most electromagnets are created by a current flowing through:
    a. Lodestones
    b. A coil
    c. A permanent magnet
    d. Ferromagnetic material

15. Positioning a permanent magnet core in the middle of the coils is called:
    a. An electromagnet
    b. A solenoid
    c. An induced current
    d. A dipole

16. Electromagnetic induction occurs when a wire is moved through a magnetic field, inducing:
    a. A stronger magnet
    b. A current
    c. Wider fields
    d. The poles to reverse

17. A current will increase in electromagnetic induction when the:
    a. Number of coils increases
    b. Speed of motion increases
    c. Strength of the magnet increases
    d. All of the above

18. The process in which one current induces another current is called:
    a. Self-induction
    (b.) Mutual induction
    c. Auto-induction

19. The process by which a magnetic field induces a current in the same wire and creates a resistance within the circuit is called:
    (a.) Self-induction
    b. Mutual induction
    c. Auto-induction

20. An electric generator produces current by rotating loops of wire through a:
    (a.) Fixed magnetic field
    b. Rotating magnetic field
    c. Auto-induced magnetic field

21. Adding slip rings and brushes to the ends of the coil in the generator allows for the production of:
    a. An alternating current
    (b.) A direct current
    c. A self-induced current

22. A motor in which the magnetic field around the coils in the center is created by a series of electromagnets rather than fixed magnets is called:
    a. An alternating-current motor
    b. A direct-current motor
    c. An induction motor

23. In transformers the electric energy in the primary coil is transformed into:
    a. Mechanical energy in the secondary coil
    b. Magnetic energy in the secondary coil
    c. Electric energy in the secondary coil

24. Transformer law states that there is a direct proportion between the ratio of wire turns on a coil and the ratio of:
    a. Voltage
    b. Ohms
    c. Amperes

25. What type of transformer has a wire wound only once around the magnetic core, and the winding is used as both the primary and secondary coils?
    a. Autotransformer
    b. Shell transformer
    c. Closed-core transformer

26. To which of the following can the inverse square law be applied?
    a. Electromagnetic radiation
    b. Magnetic fields
    c. Electric fields
    d. All of the above

Answer Key

1. a

2. d

3. a

4. b

5. b

6. a

7. d

8. c

9. b

10. c

Answers to Review

1. Charged particle, electric force, magnetic field

2. Neutral, electrons, magnetic field

3. Attract, repel, south, magnetic field

4. Lodestones, artificial permanent magnet, temporary

5. Right hand rule, same

6. Coil, permanent magnetic core, solenoid

7. Polarity, alternates, pulsing

8. Second coil, motion, magnetic, current

9. Alternating, polarity, mutual induction

10. Alternating, generator's, alternating

11. Brushes, coil, alternating

12. Voltage, high, current

13. Secondary, coils, twice, coil

14. Closed-core transformer, shell transformer, secondary

Answers to Learning Quiz

1. The primary difference between electric fields and magnetic fields is that magnetic fields attract only ferromagnetic material. An electric field exerts a force on any kind of charged particle, just as a gravitational field exerts a force on anything with mass.

2. The magnetic field of the magnet affects the spinning of electrons in a nearby metal. The electrons nearest the magnet are influenced to spin in the same direction, temporarily becoming the opposite pole of a magnet that is then attracted to the magnet.

3. The answer to this question can be determined by placing a magnet next to a compass. The experiment will show that the magnetic field close to the refrigerator magnet is stronger than the earth's, since it pulls the compass needle to it, away from the magnetic north pole of the earth.

4. An electric current creates a magnetic field in the process called induction. The opposite phenomenon, movement through a magnetic field, creates an electric current in the process called electromagnetic induction.

5. As the current alternates, what was first the north pole now becomes the south, then the north again, and so on, making a kind of pulsing in and out of the field.

6. Direct current is the kind of current produced by a battery except that it is pulsating, whereas a battery produces a steady current.

7. The word *core* refers to the ferromagnetic material around which the coils are wrapped. This material becomes magnetic along with the coils, which increases and focuses the overall magnetic field within the transformer.

Answers to Applications

1. The situation is similar to the balance of charges between electrons and protons. Even though every electron has a negative charge, most atoms are neutral because they have the same number of positive charges. Even though every electron creates a magnetic field, the fields are randomly oriented and tend to cancel each other out.

2. The answer is $\frac{1}{90}$ T. The distance of 3 mm is three times the distance of 1 mm, so the intensity diminishes by the *square* of 3, or 9. Thus the intensity is $\frac{1}{9}$ of what it is at 1 mm.

3. Tripling the coils from 75 to 225 triples the voltage induced.

4. The correct answer is six times stronger. Doubling the coils makes the current twice as strong, and tripling the speed of movement also triples the current, making a total of six times stronger.

5. The answer is 660 V, because there are three times as many turns of wire in the secondary coil, and therefore the voltage is three times as high.

6. Since the number of turns in the secondary coil is half the number in the primary coil, the voltage is also half. Therefore the voltage in the secondary coil is 110 V.

7. Just like a magnet, the movement of electrons in an electric current makes a magnetic field that affects the compass needle.

Rectification

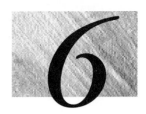

Self-Assessment Pretest

Use this pretest to assess your knowledge of the material in this module before you begin to work through the following exercises. Circle the best answer for each of the following questions. The answers to pretest questions are at the end of this module.

1. Which of the following is a benefit of using semiconductor rectifiers in x-ray equipment?
   a. They waste less energy
   b. They are less delicate
   c. There is a lower level of radiation
   d. All of the above

2. What type of current is needed inside an x-ray tube?
   a. Alternating current
   b. Direct current
   c. Both alternating and direct currents

3. The purpose of a rectifier tube is to:
   a. Increase the voltage
   b. Increase the frequency
   c. Convert alternating current to direct current
   d. Reduce the heat and energy loss

4. Which of the following is not present in a vacuum tube?
   a. Anode
   b. Cathode
   c. Filament
   d. Generator

5. Why is silicon used as the primary component of semiconductor material?
   a. It is a good conductor of electricity
   b. It has four electrons in the outer shell
   c. It does not bind with other elements
   d. It has fewer protons than electrons

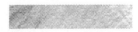

6. Which of the following is true of the n-type semiconductor?
   a. It has free electrons
   b. It has electron holes
   c. It has fixed electrons
   d. All its electrons are free

7. What are n-type and p-type semiconductors called when they are joined together?
   a. Anodes
   b. Cathodes
   c. Vacuum tubes
   d. Diodes

8. What has been developed to eliminate some of the unevenness that results from alternating current?
   a. The use of high-frequency current
   b. Three-phase generators
   c. Full-wave rectifiers
   d. All of the above

9. Which of the following is used in the production of semiconductors?
   a. Silicon
   b. Boron
   c. Phosphorus
   d. All of the above

10. What cycle current is used in most x-ray equipment to reduce the amount of rippling?
    a. 2000
    b. 60
    c. 220
    d. 110

Key Terms

Before continuing, be sure you can define the following key terms.

Anode: the positive end of a rectifier tube.

Cathode: the negative filament end of a rectifier tube.

Conduction electron: an electron that is free to move in an electron current. It is created in a semiconductor by combining silicon, which has four electrons in its outer shell, with phosphorus, which has five electrons in its outer shell. In the covalent bonding that occurs, only four of the phosphorus electrons are bonded. This leaves the fifth electron free to move.

Covalent bonding: the process in which two or more atoms are bonded by sharing some of the same electrons, which revolve around the nuclei of both or all the atoms that share them.

Diode: a device that is made by putting together an n-type and a p-type semiconductor.

Filament: a small coil of wire through which current is passed. In a vacuum-tube rectifier the filament is used to produce a stream of electrons.

Full-wave rectification: a means of using all of an alternating current that is converted to direct current. A full-wave rectifier circuit uses four rectifiers arranged in such a way that, regardless of the direction in which the alternating current is flowing, the current comes out the other end in a direct current through the full cycle.

Half-wave rectification: a process that occurs because of the cycling of alternating current. Since only half the cycle flows through, half of the current is not used but is wasted.

N-type semiconductor: a semiconductor with a free electron in its lattice. It can be made by combining silicon, which has four electrons in its outer shell, with phosphorus, which has five electrons in its outer shell. The fifth phosphorus electron is free to move. The "n" refers to the negative charge of the free electrons in the semiconductor's lattice.

P-type semiconductor: a p-type semiconductor based on a silicon lattice, which has boron atoms mixed in place of some of the silicon atoms. Since boron atoms have only three electrons in each of their outer shells, there is now a "hole" where an electron is missing. This hole is positively charged.

Rectifier: a device that converts alternating current to direct current by allowing the current to flow through it in only one direction.

Rippling: the rise and fall of the voltage in a wave. It occurs when a direct current is produced from an alternating current cycle; it falls off, moves toward reversal, and then picks back up again.

Semiconductors: a type of material "in between" an insulator and a conductor, as slush is halfway "in between" water and ice. Some current flow does occur, but with special characteristics.

Semiconductor rectifier: a rectifier that is made by putting together n-type and p-type semiconductors in a device called a diode. The semiconductor diode is a rectifier because it allows current to flow in only one direction, thus converting alternating current to direct current.

Solid-state rectifiers: a device used to create a powerful direct current from the supplied alternating current. Contemporary x-ray equipment uses solid state rectifiers.

Thermionic emission: a process that occurs when a strong current meets the resistance of a filament and causes it to become hot and emit electrons.

Vacuum tube: a device that is used to prevent oxygen from allowing a filament to burn out from the heat that it generates.

Topical Outline

The following material is covered in this module.

I. Vacuum-tube rectifiers were the first type of rectifiers developed for x-ray equipment. Vacuum-tube rectifiers are a relatively simple arrangement of components in a sealed tube.
   A. Filaments are small coils of wire through which current is passed. In a vacuum-tube rectifier the filament is used to produce a stream of electrons.
   B. An anode is the positive end of a rectifier tube, to which the electrons from the cathode are attracted.
   C. The cathode is the negative filament end of a rectifier tube, from which electrons are directed at the anode.
II. Solid-state rectifiers were developed when semiconductor technology became available. This new technology eliminated many of the problems associated with vacuum tubes.
   A. An n-type semiconductor has free electrons in its lattice. It is made by combining silicon and phosphorus, which leaves one electron per phosphorus atom that is free to move. The "n" refers to the negative charge of the free electrons.

B. A p-type semiconductor is based on a lattice of silicon and boron in which there is a "hole" because an electron is missing. This hole is positively charged.

C. A diode is made by putting together an n-type and a p-type semiconductor. This junction of the two semiconductors allows the current to flow in only one direction.

III. Rectification circuits have been developed to minimize the fluctuations in power levels that adversely affect diagnostic images.

A. Half-wave rectification occurs from the cycling of an alternating current, which results in the use of only half of a current, and therefore a pulsating on-and-off current.

B. Full-wave rectification, which uses four rectifiers, eliminates some of the problems presented by half-wave rectification. A full-wave rectifier circuit uses all of the alternating current that is being converted to direct current.

C. Three-phase generators are used to eliminate the rippling effect that is still present after full-wave rectification. These generators act to level off the cycling that is characteristic of single-phase generators.

D. High-frequency current is used in x-ray equipment to further reduce the uneven power levels. Special complex circuitry can raise the frequency to as high as 2000 cycles per second.

Review

1. When there is an electric *potential* between the filament and the plate on the other side of the tube, free *electrons* will move from the negatively-charged filament to the positively-charged *plate*. This produces an electric current.

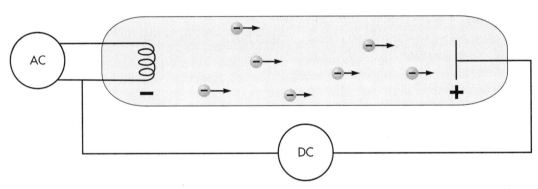

2. There are two important terms to know for the filament and metal plate inside a *rectifier* tube. The negative, filament end of the tube is called the *cathode*. The positive end is called the *anode*.

3. Metals conduct electricity well because many _electrons_ are free to move easily through the metal. You can think of the metal as almost being fluid. Insulating materials, which do not _Conduct_ electricity, are more like ice: their electrons are frozen into position and are not free to flow. _Semiconductors_ are a third type of material in between insulators and conductors, just as slush is in between water and ice. Some flow does occur, but with special characteristics.

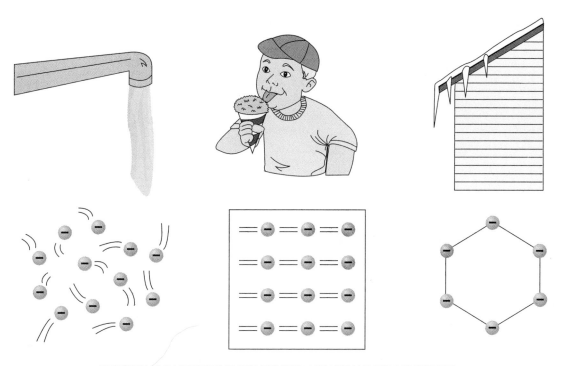

ELECTRONS IN DIFFERENT STRUCTURES ARE LIKE WATER MOLECULES:
FLUID IN WATER, SEMI-FLUID IN SLUSH, OR FROZEN IN PLACE IN ICE.

4. Shown here is a semiconductor material of mostly silicon but with some _phosphorus_ atoms in the

lattice. A phosphorus atom has __5__ electrons in its outer shell, but only four are used in the

covalent bonding with the silicon atoms. This kind of semiconductor material is called an

N-type semiconductor.

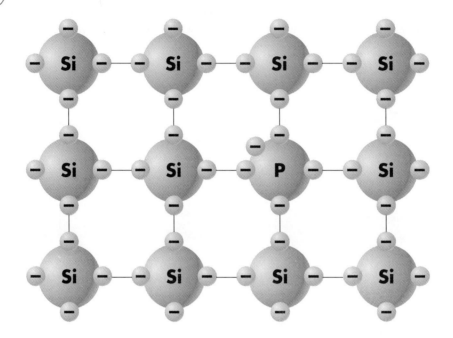

5. A p-type semiconductor is based on the silicon lattice and has _boron_ atoms mixed in place of some of the silicon atoms. Since boron atoms have only __3__ electrons in each of their outer shells, there is now a _whole_ where an electron is missing. This is _positive_ charged.

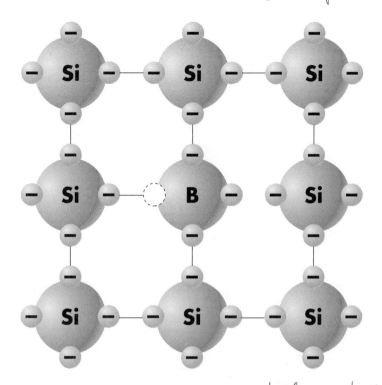

6. A semiconductor rectifier is made by putting together _N-type_ and _p-type_ semiconductors. Joined together, these semiconductors are called a _diode_.

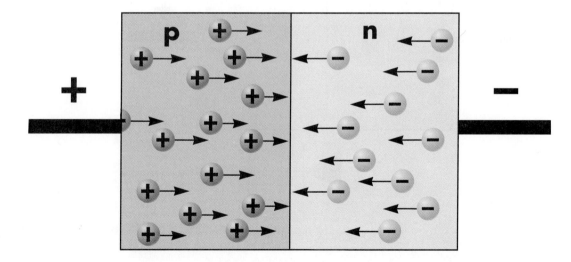

7. As shown here, an electric potential is put across a _diode_ with the positive side on the p-type semiconductor and the negative side on the n-type semiconductor. The electrons are attracted toward the _postice_ charge and move through the n-type material to the junction between the two _semiconductors_ . The _positive_ holes are attracted toward the negative charge and move through the p-type material to the junction. At the junction itself, the electrons flow into the positive _w holes_ and fill them.

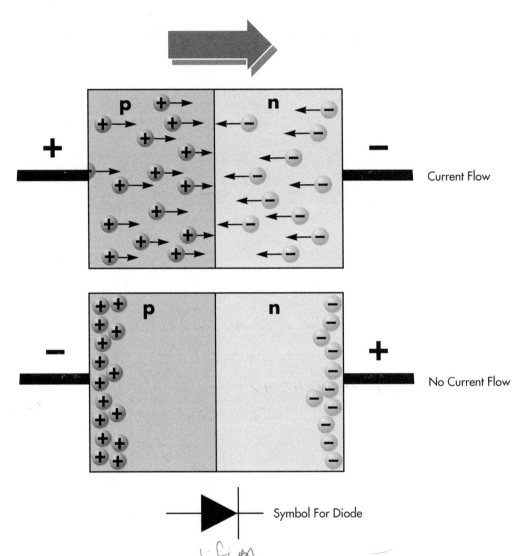

Current Flow

No Current Flow

Symbol For Diode

8. The semiconductor diode is a _rectifier_ because it allows current to flow in only one direction, thus converting _alternative_ to direct current. If the outside electric potential is an alternating current, a _direct_ current will be produced through the rectifier. It will stop the flow of current when the alternating current _reverses_. The rectifier never allows a flow in the other direction.

9. A rectifier lets only __1/2__ the cycle flow through. However, the alternating current is still flowing during the time it cannot pass through the __rectifier__, and the energy has to go some-where. It usually is wasted in producing __heat__ . In the earliest x-ray machines this heat frequently burned out the __tube__ .

10. Scientists found a way, however, to use the other half of the alternating current cycle in a __full-wave__ . This circuit uses __4__ rectifiers arranged in such a way that, regardless of the direction in which the alternating current is flowing, the current still comes out on the other end as a __direct current__ , through the full cycle.

11. In the following illustration of a full-wave rectifier, the flow of the current starts from the __positive__ side of the alternating current source, is directed by rectifier A, and emerges as a __direct current__ . The direct current flows back into the circuit through rectifier B to the __negative__ side of the alternating current.

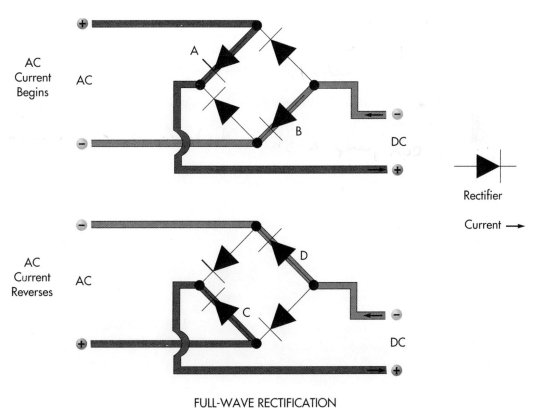

FULL-WAVE RECTIFICATION

12. The rise and fall of the _Voltage_ in a current is called "rippling." Scientists have found a way to eliminate most of this rippling and therefore to produce a steadier _dc_. This is done with three-phase generators. In these generators _3_ coils of wire are wrapped around the core of the generator in such a way that they rotate one-third of a spin apart from each other. These three coils produce three different _alternating_ currents that are in different phases, as shown here.

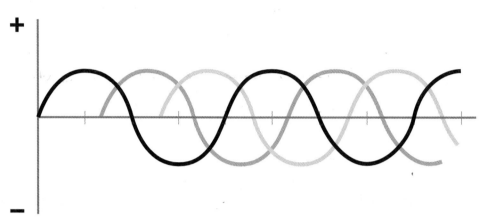

Learning Quiz

The following material is similar to the interactive exercises found in the CD-ROM version of this module operated in the "student mode." These questions will allow you to review the concepts presented in this module and will help you to gain a more complete understanding of the material.

1. If there is no wire or other conduit for the electrons in the cathode to travel to the anode, how do they cross the empty space?

    electrons can jump a short distance in a vacuum

2. Describe how covalent bonding works in semiconductor material.

in covalent bonding 2 atom share 1 electron & are bonded together

3. Why is the free electron in the n-type semiconductor free to move?

because its not bonded to other electrons

4. How does the electrostatic principle of repulsion and attraction apply to the semiconductor diode?

because opposites attract & alikes repel. the negative charge electrons are attracted to the positive hole

5. What are the advantages of using solid state diodes instead of vacuum tubes?

diodes use less energy + last longer

6. How would the rise and fall of voltage, called "rippling," affect an x-ray image?

high intensity machines have less rippling that causes constant voltage when the ripples are larger the can drop to zero + needs more energy to return to peak

7. How does the three-phase generator affect the image-making capabilities of x-ray equipment?

3 phase would be more constant

Applications

1. Why does the direct current in a rectifier always flow in the same direction?

2. Where does electric potential develop in a rectifier tube?

3. Why is a free electron created in the n-type semiconductor?

4. Why is an electron hole created in the p-type semiconductor?

because boron only has 3 electrons in its covalent bonding

5. Why are electrons attracted to the hole in p-type semiconductors?

because the hole is positively charged & the free electron on the p-type are negatively charges

6. What happens when an electric potential is put across the diode with the positive side on the p-type semiconductor and the negative side on the n-type semiconductor?

7. As is true when a diode is connected to an alternating current, what happens when the electric potential on the outside of a diode is reversed, so that the charge on the p-type side is negative and the charge on the n-type side is positive?

8. What are the disadvantages of half-wave rectification?

9. The rippling effect can cause weak currents. Why are weak currents a problem in radiography?

10. How does the three-phase generator reduce the rippling effect?

Posttest

Circle the best answer for each of the following questions. Your instructor has the correct answers.

1. What is the reason for using a semiconductor rectifier instead of a vacuum tube?
   a. It wastes less energy
   b. It's less delicate
   c. To avoid low-level radiation
   d. All of the above

2. A rectifier works by allowing current to flow through it in:
   a. One direction
   b. Both directions
   c. Alternating directions

3. To operate, the x-ray tube needs:
   a. Alternating current
   b. Direct current
   c. Both alternating and direct currents

4. What charge does the filament in a vacuum tube have?
   a. Positive
   b. Negative
   c. Neutral
   d. Both positive and negative

5. What is the positive side of a rectifier tube called?
   a. Anode
   b. Cathode
   c. Filament
   d. Transformer

6. What generates the heat that causes much of the energy of a vacuum tube to be lost?
   a. Filament
   b. Anode
   c. Transformer
   d. High voltage wires

7. What is the primary component of semiconductor material?
   a. Phosphorus
   b. Boron
   c. Silicon
   d. Tungsten

8. What type of atoms are mixed in with the p-type semiconductor?
   a. Phosphorus
   b. Boron
   c. Tungsten
   d. Lead

9. The n-type semiconductor has:
   a. A free electron
   b. Electron holes
   c. Fixed electrons
   d. All free electrons

10. A semiconductor rectifier is made by putting together n-type and p-type semiconductors. Joined together, what are these semiconductors are called?
    a. Anodes
    b. Cathodes
    c. Vacuum tubes
    d. Diodes

11. What do full-wave rectifiers use to convert an alternating current into a direct current?
    a. Four rectifiers
    b. Two alternating rectifiers
    c. Direct-current generator
    d. Single-phase generator

12. What has been developed to reduce the effects of rippling?
    a. Single-phase generators
    b. Three-phase generators
    c. Full-wave rectifiers
    d. Half-wave rectifiers

13. What is the effect of a three-phase generator?
    a. It reduces the ripple effect
    b. It reduces the energy
    c. It converts alternating current to direct current
    d. It reduces heat loss

14. How does the rippling effect produced in a current affect x-ray production?
    a. It prevents the photons from penetrating
    b. It produces low-energy x-rays that create poor images
    c. It makes the rectifier inoperative
    d. It produces double exposure images

15. In the United States, in how many cycles per second do electrons in a standard alternating current change directions?
    a. Not at all
    b. Depends on the voltage
    c. 60 times
    d. 150 times

16. What is the filament end of the rectifier tube called?
    a. Anode
    b. Cathode
    c. Diode
    d. Target plate

17. Where is the free electron known as a conduction electron found?
    a. N-type semiconductors
    b. P-type semiconductors
    c. They are emitted from diodes
    d. In silicon

18. What is the purpose of solid-state rectifiers?
    a. To prevent the filament from burning out
    b. To create direct current
    c. To level out alternating current
    d. All of the above

19. Which of the following has four electrons in its outer shell?
    a. Silicon
    b. Boron
    c. Phosphorus
    d. All of the above

20. What charge does the hole or absence of an electron have in the p-type semiconductor?
    a. Positive
    b. Negative
    c. Neutral
    d. None

21. A single rectifier tube allows:
    a. All the supplied alternating current to flow through the tube
    b. No direct current to flow through the tube
    c. Half the supplied alternating current to flow through the tube
    d. No current at all to flow through the tube

22. What is the primary negative effect of half-wave rectification?
    a. Unstable electrical energy levels
    b. Excess heat
    c. Uncontrollable levels of x-ray energy
    d. All of the above

23. From full-wave rectification is produced a:
    a. Pulsating alternating current
    b. Pulsating direct current
    c. No longer any pulsating current

24. How much of the current from an alternating current source does full-wave rectification use?
    a. None
    b. One-quarter
    c. Half
    d. All

Answer Key

1. d

2. b

3. c

4. d

5. b

6. a

7. d

8. d

9. d

10. a

Review

1. Potential, electrons, plate

2. Rectifier, cathode, anode

3. Electrons, conduct, Semiconductors

4. Phosphorus, five, covalent, n-type

5. Boron, three, hole, positively

6. N-type, p-type, diode

7. Diode, positive, semiconductors, positive, holes

8. Rectifier, alternating current, direct, reverses

9. Half, rectifier, heat, tube

10. Full-wave rectifier, four, direct current

11. Positive, direct current, negative

12. Voltage, direct current, three, alternating

Answers to Learning Quiz

1. Electrons can jump a short distance across an electric potential, inside the vacuum tube. This is like lightning passing through the air.

2. In covalent bonding, two or more atoms are bonded by sharing some of the same electrons, which revolve around the nuclei of both or all of the atoms that share them. These atoms are now stuck together as a single molecule.

3. This conduction electron is free to move because it is not bonded into the latticework of the silicon crystal. It is more like the free electrons in metal, able to conduct a current.

4. The attraction of the electrons to the positive side, and the positive holes to the negative side, is the usual electrostatic principle that similar charges repel and opposite charges attract each other.

5. Solid state diodes waste less energy in heat and are less delicate, and are therefore used in x-ray and other kinds of electric devices. Vacuum tubes also have the disadvantage of producing some low-level radiation.

6. Rippling would produce a wavy stream of x-rays, some at high intensity, some at low intensity. Effective x-ray image making depends on having control over the production of x-rays so that just enough are produced at just the right energy levels to make the ideal radiographic image.

7. Since effective image making requires predictable and constant levels of power, it is of great benefit to provide an even level of energy. With the three-phase generator, the power level would be at a more constant level at the tops of the curves. This produces x-rays at a more even energy level for more effective imaging.

Answeres to Applications

1. This is a direct current because no matter what direction the alternating current is flowing in through the filament at any moment, it is always emitting electrons and thus is always negatively charged. The electrons always move to the positive plate on the other side. Thus the alternating current in this vacuum tube rectifier has produced a direct current.

2. As the electrons are emitted from the filament, an electric potential develops between the negatively-charged filament and the metal plate at the other end, which in relation to the negative charge is positive.

3. The n-type semiconductor is made from a covalent bond between silicon and phosphorus atoms. Silicon has four electrons in its outer electron shell. A phosphorus atom has five electrons in its outer shell, but only four are used in the covalent bonding with the silicon atoms. This extra electron is therefore free to move in an electron current.

4. The p-type semiconductor is made from a covalent bond between silicon and boron atoms. Silicon has four electrons in its outer electron shell. Since boron atoms have only three electrons in each of their outer shells, there is now a "hole" where an electron is missing. This hole is positively charged.

5. Since an electron is needed to make the p-type semiconductor arrangement stable, the positively-charged hole is an electron "trap," which attracts any free conduction electron nearby.

6. The electrons are attracted toward the positive charge and move through the n-type material to the junction between the two semiconductors. The positive holes are attracted toward the negative charge and move through the p-type material to the junction. At the junction itself, the electrons flow into the positive holes and fill them.

7. All the electrons are attracted away from the junction toward the positive side of the potential, and the positive holes are similarly attracted away from the junction to the negative side of the potential. Neither positive nor negative charges are crossing the junction. In short, there is no flow through the diode at all.

8. One disadvantage of half-wave rectification is that it is not a steady flow but a pulsating on-and-off current. Second, the alternating current is still flowing during the time it cannot pass through the rectifier, and the energy has to go somewhere. It usually is wasted in producing heat. In the earliest x-ray machines this heat frequently burned out the tube.

9. Weak currents produce x-rays with lower energy, and these x-rays do not penetrate the body as well. Low-energy x-rays result in poorer images and higher radiation doses absorbed by the patient.

10. The three coils of wire in the three-phase generator are wrapped around the core of the generator in such a way that they rotate one-third of a spin apart from each other. This results in three different alternating currents being generated. Together these waves produce a more uniform current so that if you could ride only on the tops of these waves, you'd never come down to the zero point.

X-Ray Tubes and Circuits

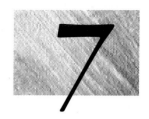

Self-Assessment Pretest

Use this pretest to assess your knowledge of the material in this module before you begin to work through the following exercises. Circle the best answer for each of the following questions. The answers to pretest questions are at the end of this module.

1. The electrons emitted from the filament in an x-ray tube ideally will:
   a. Push electrons in atoms of the anode to higher shells
   b. Turn into heat energy after hitting the anode
   c. Pass out the other end of the tube
   d. Knock electrons out of their shells in atoms of the anode

2. Which element is used in the filament to resist the effects of heat?
   a. Tungsten
   b. Iron
   c. Carbon
   d. Phosphorus

3. Electrons from the filament are concentrated toward the anode through the use of the:
   a. Filament
   b. Target
   c. Rotor
   d. Focusing cup

4. What charge is required to focus the electrons from the filament toward the anode target?
   a. Positive
   b. Negative
   c. Neutral
   d. Either positive or negative

5. Why are rotating anode targets used in some x-ray equipment?
   a. They are less fragile
   b. They are less costly
   c. They are not limited to high power settings
   d. They are less damaged from heat

6. The sharpness of an x-ray image is adversely affected by:
   a. Increasing the size of the focal spot
   b. Decreasing the size of the focal spot
   c. Decreasing the angle of the target

7. Which of the following is used in the anode cooling chart formula?
   a. Peak voltage
   b. Current
   c. Exposure time
   d. All of the above

8. Which circuit in x-ray equipment has the primary function of increasing voltage?
   a. Primary
   b. Secondary
   c. Filament

9. What is the voltage of the current supplied to x-ray equipment?
   a. 110
   b. 220
   c. 350
   d. 2000 or more

10. Which component of x-ray equipment requires a step-down transformer?
    a. Primary circuit
    b. Secondary circuit
    c. Filament circuit

Key Terms

Before continuing, be sure you can define the following key terms.

Ammeter: a device that measures current in milliamperes (mA) and shows the current flowing through the x-ray tube.

Anode: the positively-charged side of a tube, where the electrons strike a metal target and produce x-rays.

Anode cooling chart: a device used to prevent the damage that is caused by not letting an anode cool sufficiently before the tube is used again in another x-ray exposure. The anode cooling chart shows how long it takes the tube to cool from its maximum level of heat.

Autotimers: a device that controls exposure by reacting to the x-rays that actually reach the area of the photographic plate. This kind of timer can terminate the exposure when sufficient x-rays have reached the film, thus automatically accounting for differences in patient thickness.

Autotransformer: a device that raises or lowers voltage somewhat, depending on the setting used on the machine's control panel for the kilovolt peak voltage (kVp).

Cathode: the negatively-charged filament end of an x-ray tube.

Circuit breakers: a device that is included in the primary circuit to protect against short circuits and shock hazards.

Current measured in milliamps: Current measured in milliamps (mA) is one of three variables the radiographer adjusts in making an x-ray exposure.

Dual-focus tube: a device used in modern x-ray tubes that has two different filaments, one larger than the other. The larger filament produces more electrons than the smaller filament and requires a higher current.

Filament: the part of the x-ray tube that is the essential component in the filament circuit. A low voltage flowing through the filament causes the metal wire to heat up and give off electrons by the process of thermionic emission.

Focusing cup: a shell-like device behind and to the sides of the filament that helps direct the electrons from the filament in the direction of the anode.

Heel effect: a process that is caused by the angle of the target. The heel side of an x-ray beam from a tube is slightly less intense than the toe side of the beam. This occurs because the x-rays on the heel side travel through more metal than those on the toe side.

Kilovolt peak: the kilovolt (kV) level at which an x-ray exposure will be made; an adjustment the radiographer makes at the x-ray machine console; abbreviated as kVp.

Leakage radiation: a process that occurs because not all x-rays are completely absorbed by the protective housing surrounding the x-ray tube.

Line-focus principle: a process that occurs when different target angles create different size focal spots in the x-ray beam.

Main switch: an initial component in the primary circuit. When it is open, no current reaches the circuit and the machine cannot operate; when it closes, the electric current flows into the x-ray machine.

Primary circuit: a device that takes the 220 volts of the electric power supplied and increases it to the level necessary for producing x-rays in the secondary circuit.

Protective housing: a device that surrounds the x-ray tube and protects both the tube and the people nearby. The housing is lead-lined to absorb x-rays.

Rotating anode: an anode that works the same as a stationary anode (see below) in that the electron beam is focused on it and x-rays are emitted. However, to avoid the problems of heat build-up, a rotating anode turns in many revolutions per minute (rpm).

Secondary circuit: a device that begins with the secondary coil of the primary circuit's transformer. Because the secondary coil of this transformer has many more windings of wire than the primary side, the voltage is much higher. This is the kilovoltage needed to power the x-ray tube, which is also part of the secondary circuit.

Stationary anode: an anode that is fixed in place so that the electron beam always hits the same place. X-ray equipment with stationary anode tubes is used in circumstances where less heat is generated in the anode.

Step-down transformer: a device that is included in the secondary circuit to lower the voltage that reaches the filament.

Step-up transformer: a device that raises voltage to the kilovolt level needed to power the x-ray tube. A very high voltage is needed to produce x-rays.

Target: the part of the anode that is actually struck by the stream of electrons and where the x-rays are therefore produced.

Thermal capacity: the general heat limits of an x-ray tube. Too much heat over time can damage the tube, or it can instantly burn out or malfunction if it reaches too high a temperature.

Thermal stress: a result of the constant heating and cooling of the metal anode.

Timer switch: a part of the primary circuit that controls how long an x-ray tube is turned on to produce the x-ray exposure. Timer switches may be mechanical, electronic, or automatic.

Tube housing cooling chart: a device that shows how much time is needed for the housing to cool down after the maximum heat capacity has been reached.

Tube rating chart: a device that shows how the peak kilovolt level, x-ray exposure, and current measured in milliamps interact to produce tube heat. The chart also shows the maximum heat limit for a single exposure with the tube.

Tungsten: the element used in the filament of the cathode and the target part of the anode.

Window: the section of glass below the target, through which the x-ray beam emerges.

X-ray exposure: the length of exposure time used in creating a radiographic image.

X-ray tube: the final part of the secondary circuit. The high-voltage current produced by the step-up transformer and converted into a direct current by the rectifiers applies the electric potential across the anode and cathode.

Topical Outline

The following material is covered in this module.

I. The x-ray tube includes the cathode, the anode, and the protective housing that surrounds the tube.
   A. The cathode is the negatively-charged filament end of the x-ray tube.
   B. The anode is the positively-charged end of the tube, where the electrons strike the metal target and produce the x-rays.
   C. The protective housing surrounds the x-ray tube and protects both the tube and the people nearby. The housing is lead-lined to absorb x-rays.

II. X-ray tube thermal capacity is monitored by tube rating charts, anode cooling charts, and tube-housing cooling charts.
   A. Tube rating charts show how the kilovolt peak, x-ray exposure time, and current measured in milliamps interact to produce tube heat.
   B. Anode cooling charts are used to prevent the damage that is caused by not letting the anode cool sufficiently before the tube is used again in another x-ray exposure.
   C. Tube-housing cooling charts show how much time is needed for the housing to cool down after the maximum heat capacity has been reached.

III. X-ray circuitry includes the primary circuit, secondary circuit, and filament circuit.
   A. The primary circuit takes the 220-volt electric power that is supplied and increases it to the level necessary for producing x-rays in the secondary circuit.
   B. The secondary circuit begins with the secondary coil of the primary circuit's transformer and includes the x-ray tube as part of its circuit.
   C. The filament circuit includes the filament component of the x-ray tube.

Review

1. The main parts of the x-ray tube are a cathode and __anode__ . A current in the __filament__ of the

   cathode causes electrons to boil off and flow in a stream to strike the anode. These high-velocity

   electrons have __Kenetic__ energy. When they strike the metal of the anode, they penetrate atoms

   and cause them to emit __radiant__ energy.

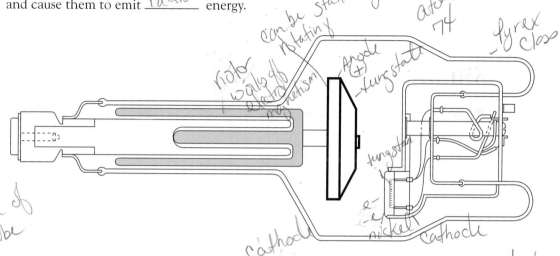

(handwritten annotations around diagram:) motor — walls of electron — magnetism — can be stationary or rotating — Anode (+) — tungstate — atomic # 74 — pyrex Class — tungsten — e- e- — nickel — Cathode — Cathode — Stator outside of tube

2. The focusing cup is positioned around the __cathode__ . Its purpose is to help direct the __electron__

   from the filament in the direction of the __Anode__. The focusing cup uses the same principle of

   __electrostatic__ repulsion.

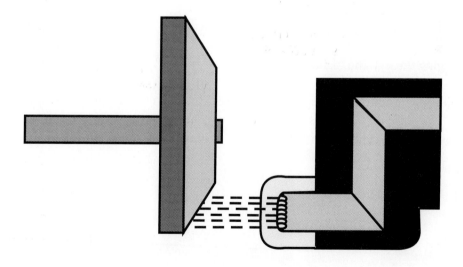

CATHODE—WITH FOCUSING CUP

3. A rotating anode works the same as a _stationary_ anode. However, instead of the electrons always striking the same spot, they strike only a small part of the target disk at any one time. The size of the focus spot stays the same, but as the anode rotates, the _target_ plate sweeps past the focal point so that the heat build-up is spread over the entire rotating anode disc, not just the one small _focal spot_

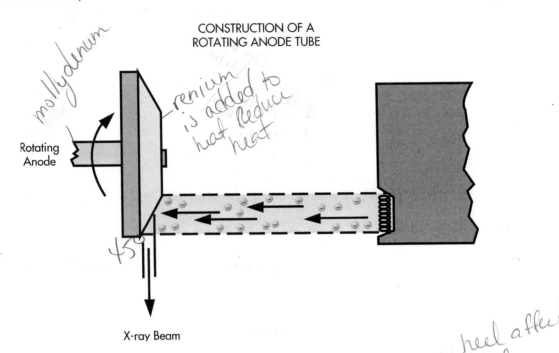

CONSTRUCTION OF A
ROTATING ANODE TUBE

Rotating
Anode

X-ray Beam

4. The shape of the anode target results in a variable x-ray beam intensity called the _line focused principle_ Compare the distance of the x-rays emerging from the heel of the path of x-rays to the distance of those emerging through the "_heel affect_." Because x-rays on the heel side travel through more metal than those on the toe side, more x-rays are _absorbed_ in the metal. Therefore the heel side of the x-ray beam from the tube is slightly _less intense_ than the toe side of the beam.

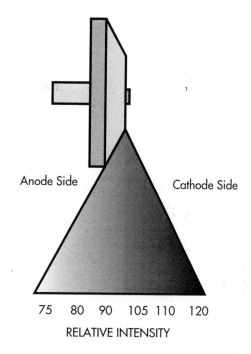

Anode Side   Cathode Side

75   80   90   105 110   120
RELATIVE INTENSITY

5. Around the x-ray tube is its protective housing, which protects both the tube and the _people_ nearby. The housing is ___lead___ -lined to absorb x-rays except those in the useful x-ray beam. This housing absorbs almost all the x-rays; those that escape the housing outside the intended useful beam are called ___leakage radiation___.

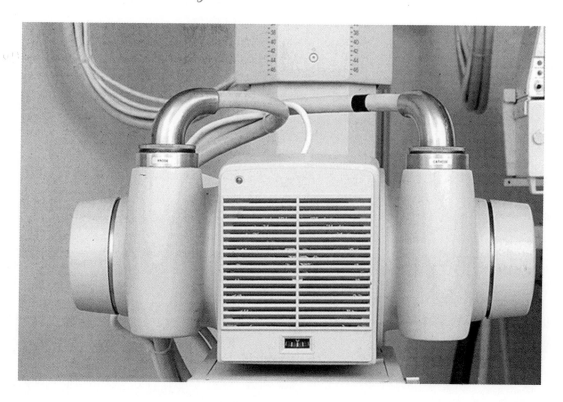

6. The limits in general of an x-ray tube are called its _thermal_ capacity. The manufacturers of x-ray

   tubes provide three different kinds of charts to help prevent exceeding that capacity. These are

   the _tube_ rating chart, the _anode cooling_ chart, and the _housing cooling_ chart.

7. Using the tube rating chart shown, consider two different exposures. Note the dot on the chart

   that represents an exposure of 0.1 second at 150 mA. This dot is beneath the 90 kVp curve,

   meaning that this exposure is _safe_ for the tube. Now consider the second dot, which repre-

   sents an exposure of 0.5 seconds at 150 mA. This dot is _above_ the 90 kVp curve, meaning

   that this exposure may dangerously overheat the tube and should not be made.

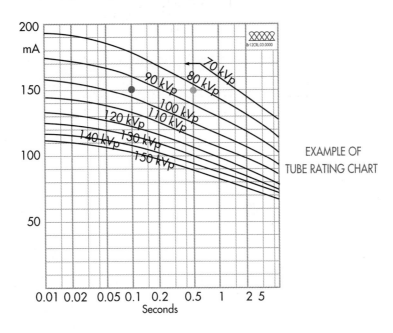

EXAMPLE OF
TUBE RATING CHART

8. The tube rating chart is used to determine whether the specified _exposure_ is safe or unsafe. With a current of 130 milliamps, a peak voltage of 110 kilovolts, and an exposure time of 0.5 seconds, the exposure is _above_ the safety curve line. That exposure would exceed the tube's _thermal_ capacity.

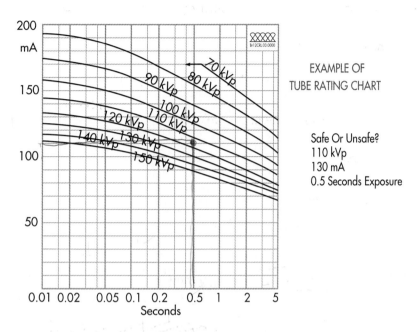

9. The anode cooling chart is used to prevent damage caused by not letting the _anode_ cool sufficiently before the tube is used again in another x-ray _exposure_. The anode cooling chart shows
how long it takes the tube to cool from its _max_ level of heat. As the formula shows, heat
units are calculated by multiplying the peak _voltage_ by the current by the exposure time in
seconds.

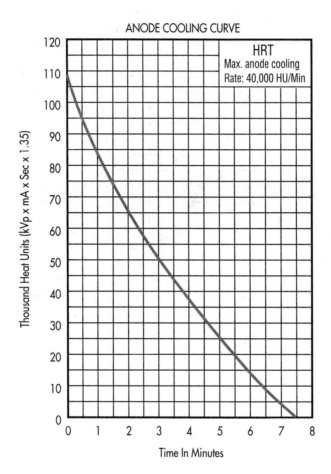

heat units = KVp X mA X Sec

10. The anode cooling chart can be used to calculate cooling time even when the heat level is not at the tube's _capacity_. In this example, an exposure of 100 _kvp_ at 200 milliamps for 2 seconds produces 54,000 _heat_ units. That is the point on the curve at which the tube would have _cooled_ down from its maximum level after 2.5 minutes.

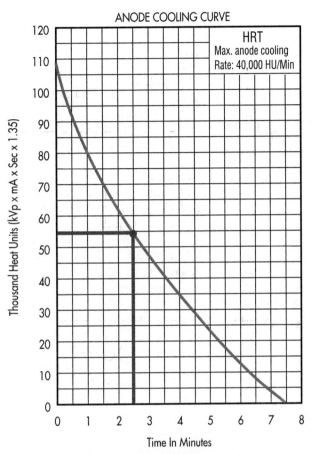

ANODE COOLING CURVE

HRT
Max. anode cooling
Rate: 40,000 HU/Min

Thousand Heat Units (kVp x mA x Sec x 1.35)

Time In Minutes

Example: 100 kVp x 200 mA x 2 seconds
x 1.35 (specific tube factor)
= 54,000 HU

11. The x-ray tube itself is the final part of the _secondary_ circuit. The high-voltage current produced by the _step-up transform_ and converted into a _DC_ current by the rectifiers applies the electric potential across the anode and cathode.

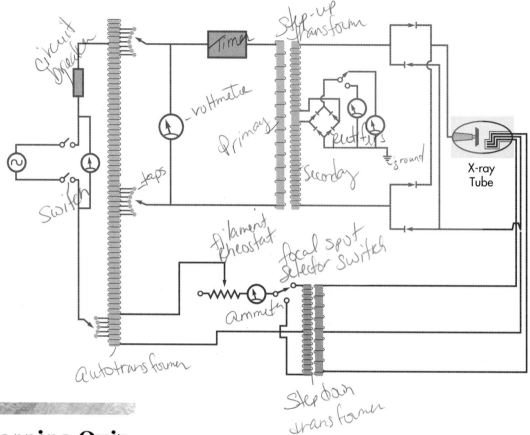

Learning Quiz

The following material is similar to the interactive exercises found in the CD-ROM version of this module operated in the "student mode." These questions will allow you to review the concepts presented in this module and will help you to gain a more complete understanding of the material.

1. Why is the control of voltage one of the key factors in x- ray equipment?

2. What two different currents flow into the cathode?

3. What is the trade-off between the angle of the anode target and the focal spot?

4. What factors contribute to the heel effect besides the angle of the anode target?

5. Besides telling you when the anode is completely cooled or has reached its maximum capacity, what will the anode cooling chart allow you to calculate?

6. When might the anode cooling chart calculations not be needed?

7. How is a special kind of spinning top used to test timers?

8. Why is controlling the milliamp (mA) current flowing to the filament critical in radiography?

Applications

1. What is the effect of the shell from which an atom's electron was knocked out?

2. Why is tungsten used in the anode of the x-ray tube?

3. What is the principle behind the focusing cup's ability to direct electrons to the anode?

4. How can radiographers use the heel effect to advantage when positioning a patient relative to the x-ray tube?

5. What three charts are used to help prevent exceeding the thermal capacity of the tube?

6. What three factors does the tube rating chart use to determine the thermal limits of the tube?

7. What will the formula kilovolts times milliamps times seconds times the specific tube factor tell a radiographer?

Posttest

Circle the best answer for each of the following questions. Your instructor has the correct answers.

1. Rectification is necessary to convert the supplied alternating current into a high-powered direct current to power the:
   a. X-ray tube
   b. Step-down transformer
   c. Anode
   d. Transformer

2. X-rays are produced when high-energy electrons strike the atoms of the:
   a. Anode
   b. X-ray tube
   c. Cathode
   d. All of the above

3. A photon of energy that is useful in producing an x-ray image is released each time an electron:
   a. Jumps up a shell
   b. Falls down a shell
   c. Hits another electron
   d. Hits the nucleus

4. Electrons in the outermost shell from the nucleus have:
   a. The greatest binding energy
   b. The least binding energy
   c. No binding energy
   d. The same binding energy as all other shells

5. Which element is used in the filament of the cathode?
   a. Tungsten
   b. Iron
   c. Carbon
   d. Phosphorus

6. Electrons boiling off the filament are directed by the:
   a. Filament
   b. Target
   c. kVp
   d. Focusing cup

7. What is the charge of the focusing cup?
   a. Positive
   b. Negative
   c. Neutral
   d. It alternates between positive and negative

8. What is the name of the anode in an x-ray tube in which the focused electron beam always strikes the same place?
   a. Stationary anode
   b. Rotating anode
   c. Static anode
   d. Target anode

9. What element is used for the anode target?
   a. Copper
   b. Tungsten
   c. Boron
   d. Aluminum

10. What element is used to conduct heat away from the anode target?
    a. Copper
    b. Tungsten
    c. Boron
    d. Aluminum

11. The primary problem with stationary anode targets is that they are:
    a. Fragile
    b. More costly
    c. Limited to high power settings
    d. Damaged by heat

12. What was developed to reduce the heat build-up caused by electrons hitting the same spot on a target?
    a. Cryonics elements
    b. Rotating anodes
    c. Rotating cathodes
    d. Replaceable targets

13. What directs the electron beam that strikes the target out of the bottom of the tube?
    a. A focusing cup
    b. The angle of the anode target
    c. The angle of the cathode
    d. The anode rotor

14. The sharpness of an x-ray image can be increased by:
    a. Increasing the size of the focal spot
    b. Decreasing the size of the focal spot
    c. Increasing the angle of the target

15. While the best x-ray images come from small focal spots, they create a problem of:
    a. Increased danger from radiation
    b. Burning out the filament
    c. Heating the target up too much
    d. All of the above

16. The heel side of the x-ray beam is:
    a. Stronger than the toe side
    b. Weaker than the toe side
    c. Weaker on stationary anodes but the same on rotating anodes
    d. The same as the toe side

17. The intensity of the heel effect depends on:
    a. The angle of the target
    b. The distance between the film and the x-ray tube
    c. The size of the radiographic film used
    d. All of the above

18. Which of the following is not a chart used to help prevent exceeding the thermal capacity of the x-ray tube?
    a. Anode cooling chart
    b. Tube rating chart
    c. Tube-housing cooling chart
    d. Cathode cooling chart

19. What factor does the tube rating chart use?
    a. Kilovolt peak
    b. X-ray exposure time
    c. Current measured in milliamps
    d. All of the above

20. The anode cooling chart formula is calculated by multiplying the peak voltage by the current by the:
    a. Room temperature
    b. Anode temperature
    c. Exposure time
    d. Lapsed exposure time

21. What is the main function of the primary circuit?
    a. To open and close the circuit
    b. To increase voltage
    c. To convert alternating current to direct current

22. What control is used to raise or lower the voltage in the primary circuit?
    a. The kVp selector
    b. The keV selector
    c. The mA selector

23. The rectifier circuit is located in:
    a. The primary circuit
    b. The secondary circuit
    c. The filament circuit
    d. All of the above

24. What level of voltage flows through the filament of the x-ray tube?
    a. High
    b. Low
    c. Both high and low

25. What controls the filament circuit?
    a. The kVp selector
    b. The mA selector
    c. The focal spot selector

26. The x-ray tube current is controlled by the:
    a. Filament
    b. Anode
    c. Primary circuit
    d. Secondary circuit

Answer Key

Answers to Pretest

1. d

2. a

3. d

4. b

5. d

6. a

7. d

8. a

9. b

10. c

Answers to Review

1. Anode, filament, kinetic, electromagnetic or x-ray

2. Cathode, electrons, anode, electrostatic

3. Stationary, target, focal point

4. Heel effect, toe, absorbed, less intense

5. People, lead, leakage radiation

6. Thermal, tube, anode cooling, tube-housing cooling

7. Safe, above

8. Exposure, above, thermal

9. Anode, exposure, maximum, voltage

10. Capacity, kilovolts or kVp, heat, cooled

11. Secondary, step-up transformer, direct

Answers to Learning Quiz

1. Voltage is one of the key factors that determine the velocity of the electrons and thus their kinetic energy.

2. One low-voltage current is the filament current that causes the filament to heat up. The other current creates the electric potential that repels the electrons from the cathode and attracts them to the anode.

3. The angle of the anode target also determines the focal spot size of the x-ray beam. There is a kind of trade-off here in the design of the anode. The greater the angle, the more surface area is struck by the electrons, thus spreading the heat over a greater area. But the larger angle also increases the focal spot size, which decreases the sharpness of the image. Anode angles are therefore set at a point in between the extremes, for sharpness of detail without overheating.

4. New x-ray equipment has been designed to minimize the heel effect, although it is often still present. The intensity of the effect can depend on factors such as the distance between the film and the x-ray tube and the size of the radiographic film used.

5. In reality, you might seldom allow the tube to reach the full capacity, nor can you always wait the amount of time needed for the tube to cool completely. Thus this chart also lets you calculate when it is safe to make another exposure after the first, or whether partial cooling might be needed.

6. New x-ray machines have automatic safeguards to prevent overheating of the x-ray tube, so that these calculations are not always needed. Follow the protocol for the x-ray machines in your particular setting.

7. A radiograph made with a synchronized spinning top is sometimes used to test the timer. The amount of film exposed by x-rays passing through a hole in the spinning top indicates the length of the exposure.

8. Controlling the filament current controls the tube current. Even a small change in the milliamp (mA) current flowing through the filament produces a change in the temperature of the filament and affects how many electrons are emitted to be rapidly driven at the anode. For example, an increase of only 1 mA in the filament current can increase the tube current by as much as 200 mA as many more electrons are emitted and flow in the beam to the anode.

Answers to Applications

1. The energy of an x-ray photon depends in part on from which shell the atom's electron was knocked out. Electrons in the innermost shell (closest to the nucleus) have the greatest binding energy.

2. The element tungsten is used in x-ray tubes for several reasons. Tungsten has 74 electrons, and the binding energy of the two electrons in the innermost shell is very high. X-ray photons that are emitted when these electrons are knocked out of this shell have much energy and are most effective for producing diagnostic x-ray images.

3. The focusing cup uses the principle of electrostatic repulsion. The strong negative charge of the cup pushes the electrons away from the cup and therefore in toward each other, packing them together into a tighter beam.

4. If a body area of varying thickness is to be imaged, the thinner part of the body can be placed in the less intense part of the x-ray beam (the heel part, on the anode side of the tube), and the thicker part of the body in the more intense part of the beam (toward the cathode). This will give a more uniform image.

5. The tube rating chart, the anode cooling chart, and the housing cooling chart.

6. The kilovolt peak at which the x-ray exposure will be made, the length of the x-ray exposure, and the x-ray tube current measured in milliamps.

7. This is the formula used in the anode cooling curve.

Production and Characteristics of Radiation

Self-Assessment Pretest

Use this pretest to assess your knowledge of the material in this module before you begin to work through the following exercises. Circle the best answer for each of the following questions. The answers to pretest questions are at the end of this module.

1. Of the three characteristics of x-rays, which does not contribute beneficially to the formation of an x-ray image?
   a. Absorption
   b. Penetration
   c. Scatter

2. Which of these units of measurement refers to the measure of intensity of x-ray radiation?
   a. A rad
   b. A rem
   c. A roentgen (R)

3. What is the equivalent of the SI unit seivert(Sv)?
   a. A rad
   b. A rem
   c. An electron volt (eV)
   d. A roentgen

4. What does the kilovolt peak (kVp) setting control?
   a. The focus of the image
   b. The kinetic energy of projectile electrons
   c. The degree of filtration
   d. The rads

5. Which of the following has the greatest binding energy?
   a. K shell
   b. L shell
   c. M shell
   d. N shell

6. As electrons are directed at the anode, most of the electrons:
   a. Miss the anode
   b. Hit other electrons
   c. Result in bremsstrahlung x-rays
   d. Result in characteristic x-rays

7. Which of the following controls how many projectile electrons pass from the cathode to the anode?
   a. The milliampere (mA) setting
   b. The kiloelectron volt (keV) setting
   c. The kVp setting
   d. The filtration controls

8. Filtration affects the x-ray beam by:
   a. Decreasing the quantity of x-rays
   b. Increasing the average energy of x-rays
   c. Decreasing the low-level x-rays
   d. All of the above
   e. None of the above

9. Which of the following affect the clarity of the diagnostic image?
   a. Classical scattering, pair production, and photodisintegration
   b. Photoelectric interaction, Compton scattering, and classical scattering
   c. Photoelectric interaction, classical scattering, and pair production
   d. Compton scattering, pair production, and photodisintegration

10. To reduce film fogging, Compton scattering should be:
    a. Maximized
    b. Minimized
    c. Neither; it doesn't affect film fogging

Key Terms

Before continuing, be sure you can define the following key terms.

Absorption: the process by which x-ray photons are taken in by the body as a result of the photoelectric effect. These photons do not pass through the body to strike the film. Therefore the areas of the body that absorb the most x-rays show up on the x-ray film image as clear or white.

Added filtration: the use of filters, such as aluminum plates positioned in the path of the beam, to remove additional low-energy x-rays that are of no value for imaging.

Annihilation event: a process that occurs in pair production. The positron that is created in pair production travels until it strikes an electron, with which it interacts. The proton and electron are converted into two x-ray photons that radiate out of the atom.

Attenuation: the process by which x-ray photons are absorbed and scattered and therefore removed from the x-ray beam as it passes through a body.

Barium: an element that generally absorbs x-rays and also is used as a contrast medium in some kinds of x-ray studies.

Bremsstrahlung radiation: the result occurring when a projectile electron enters an atom in the metal of the anode and does *not* strike any of that atom's electrons but continues toward the center of the atom and comes near the nucleus. As the electron nears the nucleus it slows down and loses kinetic energy, which takes the form of a photon of x-ray energy being released.

Characteristic x-ray: the result that occurs when the absence of an electron in an inner shell is immediately "corrected" in the atom by another electron jumping down to fill its place. An x-ray photon is released in this interaction.

Classical scattering: a process that is most likely to occur with low-energy x-rays (below 10 keV). When a photon from such an x-ray enters an atom, it does not have enough energy to knock out an electron and cause Compton scattering. Instead, the photon's energy causes a momentary state of excitation in the atom, a higher state of energy. This process is also called coherent, or unmodified, scattering.

Coherent scattering: a process that is most likely to occur with low-energy x-rays (below 10 keV). When a photon from such an x-ray enters an atom, it does not have enough energy to knock out an electron and cause Compton scattering. Instead, the photon's energy causes a momentary state of excitation in the atom, a higher state of energy. This process is also called classical, or unmodified, scattering.

Compton scattering: a process that is most likely to occur with x-rays in the energy range of 30 to 50 keV. The photon of the x-ray knocks an electron out of the atom that it strikes, but not all of its energy is absorbed by the interaction.

Differential absorption: the general characteristic of producing x-ray images with some structures that are radiopaque and some that are radiolucent. It is called *differential* because different body structures absorb x-rays to different extents.

Electron volt: a measure of the energy of a moving electron or x-ray photon; abbreviated as eV. An electron has 1 eV when it is accelerated by an electric potential of 1 volt (V).

Film fog: a blurring that occurs when x-ray photons strike the film in random locations.

Filtration: a means by which radiologic technologists control the quantity and quality of the x-ray beam.

Hardening the x-ray beam: the result of an increase in average x-ray energy caused by filtration.

Inherent filtration: the process by which low-level x-rays are filtered out by the glass window of the x-ray tube as the x-ray beam passes through it.

Intensity: a characteristic of a beam dependent on both quality and quantity; increasing either will raise the intensity.

kVp setting: a setting that controls the electric potential difference between the cathode and the anode. Higher kVp settings give the projectile electrons greater kinetic energy and produce a beam with x-rays of greater quantity and quality.

Pair production: a process that occurs only with very high-energy photons. A photon with an energy of at least 1022 keV (or 1.02 MeV) can penetrate through the electron shells of the atom to reach the nucleus. This energy is then converted into the production of an electron and a positron.

Penetration: the process by which x-ray photons are transmitted through the body and reach the radiographic film. If no x-ray photons penetrated the body, no image would result.

Photodisintegration: the process that occurs when x-rays with extremely high energy (above 7 MeV) strike the nucleus of the atom and make it unstable. To become stable again, this radioactive nucleus ejects a nuclear particle, such as a proton, neutron, or alpha particle.

Photoelectric interaction: the process that occurs when the energy of an incident x-ray photon is absorbed by the atom it strikes, and an electron is ejected from the inner shell of that atom.

Photoelectron: an electron that is ejected during the process of photoelectric interaction.

Positron: a positively-charged electron.

Probability: the likelihood that certain types of interactions will occur in certain situations.

Projectile electron: an electron that is produced inside an x-ray tube when electrons from the cathode strike the atoms of the anode. The kinetic energy of these electrons knocks an electron out of the atom that is struck. When an electron in a higher orbital shell falls down to replace the electron bumped out, an x-ray photon is produced.

Quality: the average energy level of x-rays in a beam.

Rad: the unit that measures the x-ray radiation energy absorbed in the body. The SI unit is the gray (Gy). Both units measure the amount of energy absorbed per unit of mass (kg).

Radiolucent: the quality of a structure that is less dense and therefore has a lower probability of absorption.

Radiopaque: the quality of a structure that is more dense and therefore absorbs x-rays more readily.

Rem: a unit that is an acronym from the words *radiation equivalent man*. It is a measure of radiation exposure in occupational settings: the amount of radiation absorbed by those who work around it. The equivalent SI unit is the seivert (Sv).

Roentgen: the unit that is used to measure the intensity of radiation; abbreviated as R. It takes 1R of radiation energy to ionize a certain number of atoms in a certain volume of air. An x-ray beam with an output measured at twice the roentgen level of another beam will be twice as intense.

Scatter: the process in which x-ray photons strike the film in random locations, producing an overall characteristic called film fog. It results from Compton scattering and classical scattering.

Secondary x-ray: the result that occurs when an electron from a higher shell jumps down to fill the place of an absent electron in an inner shell. This jump produces an x-ray photon.

Unmodified scattering: a process that is most likely to occur with low-energy x-rays (below 10 keV). When a photon from such an x-ray enters an atom, it does not have enough energy to knock out an electron and cause Compton scattering. Instead, the photon's energy causes a momentary state of excitation in the atom, a higher state of energy. This process is also called classical, or coherent, scattering.

Topical Outline

The following material is covered in this module.

I. X-ray production can take one of two forms when a projectile electron strikes an atom.

    A. Characteristic radiation occurs when the absence of an electron in an inner shell is immediately "corrected" in the atom by another electron falling down to fill its place. An x-ray photon is released in this interaction.

    B. Bremsstrahlung radiation occurs when a projectile electron enters an atom in the metal of the anode and does not strike any of that atom's electrons but continues toward the center of the atom and comes near the nucleus. There is a loss of kinetic energy, from which an x-ray photon is released.

II. There are five types of interactions of x-rays with matter: photoelectric interaction, Compton scattering, and classical scattering all affect the x-ray image; pair production and photodisintegration interactions generally do not.

    A. Photoelectric interaction occurs as the energy of the incident x-ray photon is absorbed by the atom it strikes, and an electron is ejected from the inner shell of that atom.

    B. Compton scattering interaction occurs when an x-ray photon knocks an electron out of the atom that it strikes, but not all of its energy is absorbed by this.

C. Classical scattering occurs when a photon enters an atom but does not have enough energy to knock out an electron. Instead, the photon's energy causes a momentary state of excitation in the atom, a higher state of energy.

D. Pair production occurs only with very high energy photons that can penetrate through the electron shells of the atom to reach the nucleus. This energy is then converted into the production of an electron and a positron.

E. Photodisintegration occurs when x-rays with extremely high energy strike the nucleus of the atom and make it unstable. To become stable again, this nucleus ejects a nuclear particle, such as a proton, neutron, or alpha particle.

III. Beam characteristics are crucial in determining the best settings for producing a diagnostic image.

A. Penetration occurs when the x-rays are transmitted through the body and reach the radiographic film.

B. Absorption occurs when x-ray photons are taken in by the body as a result of the photoelectric effect. These photons do not pass through the body to strike the film.

C. Scatter results in x-ray photons striking the film in random locations, producing the overall characteristic called film fog.

IV. Units of measurements for x-ray radiation include the roentgen, rem, rad, and electron volt.

A. Roentgen (R) measures the intensity of radiation.

B. Rem measures radiation exposure in occupational settings, or the amount of radiation absorbed by those who work around it.

C. Rad measures absorbed radiation.

D. Electron volt (eV) measures the energy of a moving electron or x-ray photon.

Review

1. In characteristic radiation the _____ electron strikes an atom and knocks an electron out of its orbit. This leaves the atom in an _____ state. An electron from a _____ orbit then moves down into the space left by the electron bumped out. In so doing, it gives off a _____ of x-ray radiation.

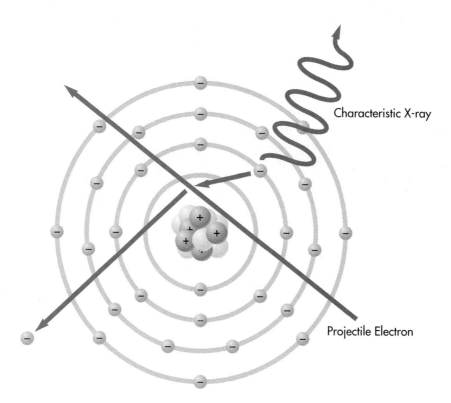

Characteristic X-ray

Projectile Electron

2. This illustration shows the innermost two electron shells, the _____ and L shells. A electron is knocked out of the K shell, and an electron from the _____ shell falls down to fill the empty space. The energy of the x-ray resulting from the fall of the L-shell electron to the K shell is calculated as the difference in _____ between the two. This interaction in the tungsten atom produces an _____ with the energy of 58.5 keV.

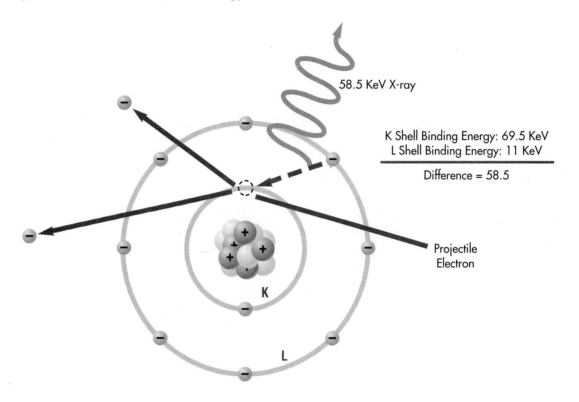

58.5 KeV X-ray

K Shell Binding Energy: 69.5 KeV
L Shell Binding Energy: 11 KeV

Difference = 58.5

Projectile
Electron

K

L

3. K shell electrons are not always replaced by electrons from the _____ shell. Electrons from shells farther out may also jump down to fill the empty space. The binding energy of electrons in shells farther out becomes progressively _____ . Therefore the x-ray energy is _____ if electrons from those shells replace the removed K shell electron.

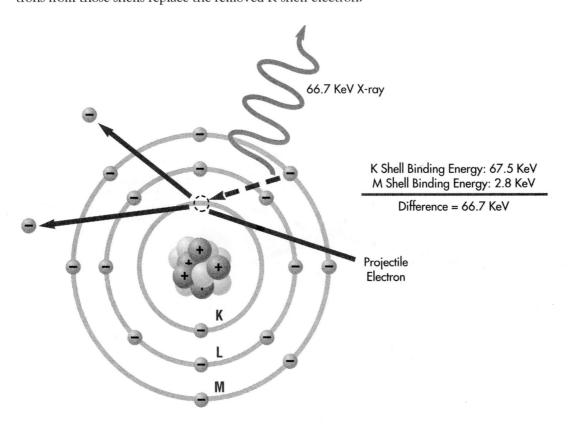

66.7 KeV X-ray

K Shell Binding Energy: 67.5 KeV
M Shell Binding Energy: 2.8 KeV
_____
Difference = 66.7 KeV

Projectile
Electron

K

L

M

4. The amount of energy in the x-ray photon depends on the original _____ energy of the projectile electron and the _____ in this energy, which in turn depends on how close the electron passes to the nucleus. The electron can give up all of its kinetic energy for _____ energy, part of its kinetic energy for lower x-ray energy, no kinetic energy at all for x-ray energy, or any amount in between.

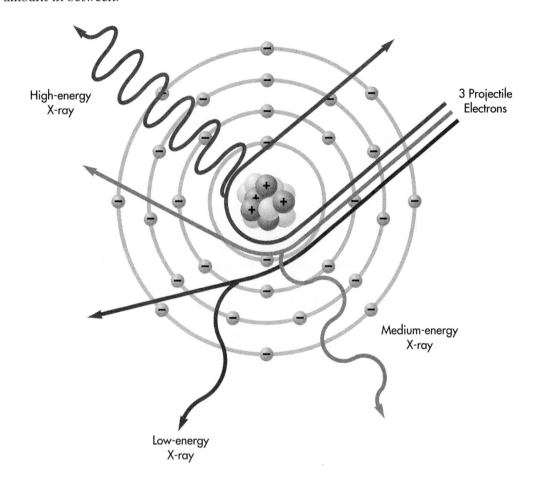

5. The height of the curve in this graph shows the _____ of x-rays at the different energy levels. The energy level of x-rays in the beam is shown on the horizontal axis; the average energy level is referred to as the _____ of the beam. The intensity of the beam depends on both quality and quantity; increasing either will raise the _____ of the beam.

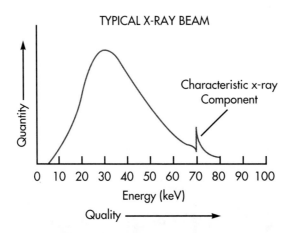

6. The mA setting for the x-ray tube current controls how many _____ pass from the cathode to the _____. Increasing the number of electrons will increase the number of x-rays produced. If the _____ setting remains the same, however, the increased number of electrons will still have the same energy levels, and the quality of the beam will not _____ even though the quantity does.

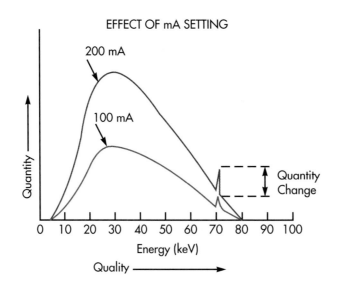

7. The use of filtration of the x-ray beam is another way that radiologic technologists control the

_____ and _____ of the x-ray beam. Inherent filtration occurs as the x-ray beams pass

through the _____ of the x-ray tube. Added filtration removes additional _____ x-rays that

are of no value for imaging because they do not have enough energy to _____ the body.

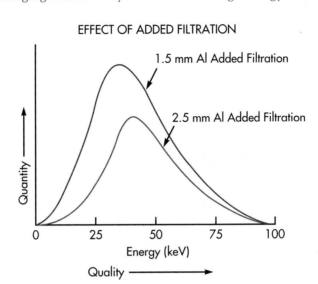

8. In the photoelectric interaction, the energy of the incident x-ray _____ is absorbed by the atom it strikes, and an electron is ejected from the _____ shell of that atom. The kinetic energy of the ejected electron, called a _____ , equals the energy of the incident x-ray minus the _____ energy of the electron that is ejected.

PHOTOELECTRIC INTERACTION

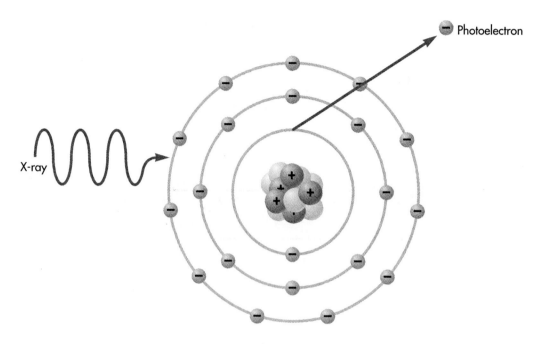

9. In the Compton scattering interaction, the x-ray photon knocks an _____ out of the atom that it strikes, but not all of its energy is _____ by this. Outer-shell electrons have lower _____ energy and thus can be knocked out of the atom without the x-ray photon losing all its energy. With the electron missing from the atom it becomes an _____.

COMPTON SCATTERING

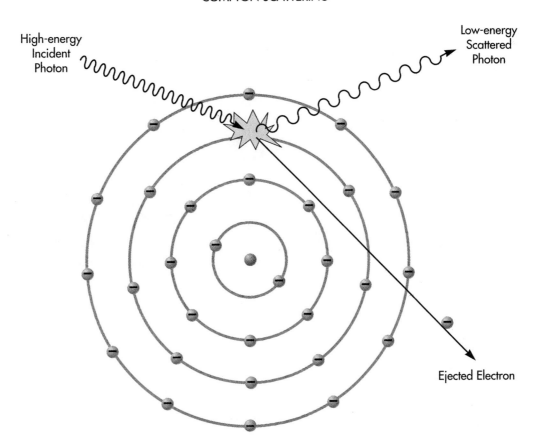

High-energy
Incident
Photon

Low-energy
Scattered
Photon

Ejected Electron

10. Classical scattering is most likely to occur with _____ x-rays below 10 keV. When a photon from such an x-ray enters an atom, it does not have enough energy to knock out an _____ and cause Compton scattering. Instead, the photon's energy causes a momentary state of _____ in the atom, a higher state of energy.

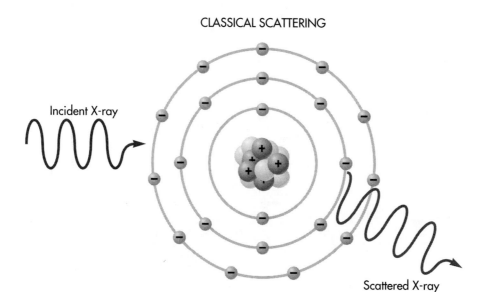

CLASSICAL SCATTERING

Incident X-ray

Scattered X-ray

11. In pair production a photon can penetrate through the electron shells of an atom to reach the

_____ . This energy is then converted into the production of an electron and a _____ ,

which is a positively-charged _____ . This travels until it strikes an electron, with which it

interacts in what is called an _____ event.

PAIR PRODUCTION

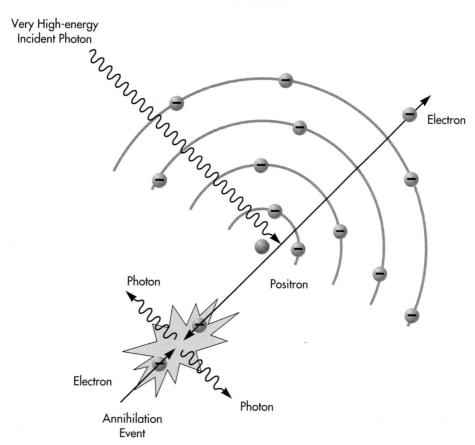

12. One last type of interaction between x-rays and _____ is called photodisintegration. X-rays with extremely _____ energy (above 7 MeV) strike the nucleus of the atom and make it _____ . To become stable again, this nucleus ejects a nuclear particle, such as a _____ , neutron, or alpha particle. This is photodisintegration.

PHOTODISINTEGRATION

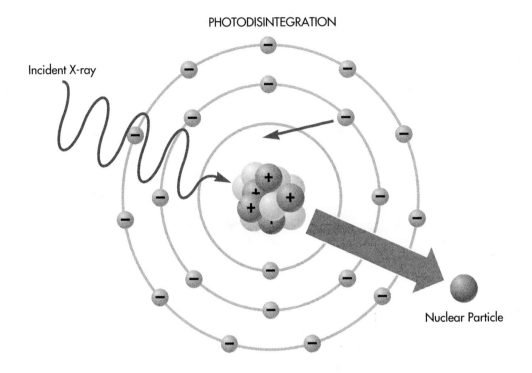

Incident X-ray

Nuclear Particle

Learning Quiz

The following material is similar to the interactive exercises found in the CD-ROM version of this module operated in the "student mode." These questions will allow you to review the concepts presented in this module and will help you to gain a more complete understanding of the material.

1. In the electromagnetic spectrum, what is above the highest energy x-rays?

2. Why does the level of x-ray energy vary from electron shell to electron shell?

3. Do the shells of all atoms have the same electron binding energy?

4. Why are there fewer high-energy characteristic x-rays than low-energy characteristic x-rays?

5. What occurs in the atoms of the body that can result in an ion from a photoelectric interaction changing or altering DNA?

6. When are higher-energy photons that may result in pair production used?

Applications

1. If an electron is knocked out of the K shell, would an electron jump from the L or the M shell provide more x-ray energy?

2. What is the M-shell binding energy if the K-shell binding energy is 69.5 and an x-ray of 66.7 keV is produced?

3. Why is a photon emitted during the bremsstrahlung interaction if the electron does not hit another electron?

4. Why does increasing the kVp setting beyond a certain point reduce the usefulness of the beam?

5. The mA setting for the x-ray tube current controls how many projectile electrons pass from the cathode to the anode. What occurs if the mA setting is increased and the kVp setting remains the same?

6. How does filtration increase the quality of an x-ray beam?

7. How can the ionization that may result from Compton scattering result in biological effects?

8. Why must a radiologic technologist be shielded?

9. What four units of measurement are used to measure x-ray radiation?

Posttest

Circle the best answer for each of the following questions. Your instructor has the correct answers.

1. Above the highest energy x-rays in the electromagnetic spectrum are:
   a. Alpha rays
   b. Beta rays
   c. Gamma rays
   d. Ultraviolet rays

2. What happens to the binding energy of an electron that is knocked out of its shell?
   a. It is released as a photon
   b. It causes a higher-level electron to move down
   c. It is released when it is knocked out of the shell
   d. All of the above

3. To knock an electron out of its shell, the kinetic energy of a projectile electron must be:
   a. At least equal to the binding energy of the electron
   b. Less than the binding energy of the electron
   c. Greater than the binding energy of the electron
   d. None of the above; kinetic energy is irrelevant

4. Which of the following has the highest approximate characteristic x-ray energy levels?
   a. K-shell interaction
   b. L-shell interaction
   c. M-shell interaction
   d. N-shell interaction

5. Assume the binding energy of an L-shell electron is 12 and that of an M shell is 2. What is the x-ray energy that results from the fall of the electron from the M shell to the L shell?
   a. 24
   b. 14
   c. 10
   d. 6

6. Which electron shells produce x-ray energy that is of no value for diagnostic imaging?
   a. K shell
   b. Shells L to N
   c. Shells greater than N
   d. All shells have diagnostic value

7. Which of the following influences whether a projectile electron strikes another electron?
   a. Chance
   b. Other electrons
   c. The nucleus
   d. All of the above

8. How does a projectile electron lose its energy in the bremsstrahlung interaction?
   a. By striking another electron
   b. By striking the nucleus
   c. By striking photons
   d. By being slowed by the force of attraction

9. How much kinetic energy may be transformed into x-ray energy during a bremsstrahlung interaction?
   a. All
   b. Only a portion
   c. None
   d. All of the above

10. When the voltage of an x-ray tube is set in the range of 100 to 150 kVp, most of the x-rays are:
    a. Characteristic
    b. Bremsstrahlung
    c. Higher level
    d. High-intensity

11. The average energy of x-rays in a beam is referred to as:
    a. Intensity
    b. Quality
    c. Quantity

12. What does the mA setting control?
    a. Number of projectile electrons
    b. Voltage
    c. Angle of the anode
    d. Distance between the anode and cathode

13. What will happen if the kVp setting remains the same and the mA setting is increased?
    a. The quality of the beam increases
    b. The quantity of photons decreases
    c. The electrons will have the same energy levels
    d. All of the above

14. How does hardening of the x-ray beam occur?
    a. By changing the kVp setting
    b. By filtration
    c. By changing the mA setting
    d. All of the above

15. As an x-ray beam passes through glass or aluminum plates, what happens to the overall energy level of the x-ray beam?
    a. It stays the same
    b. It decreases
    c. It increases
    d. It is stopped

16. When the x-ray photon reaches some material, what interaction may occur?
    a. The energy may be momentarily absorbed
    b. The energy may be totally absorbed
    c. There may be no interaction at all
    d. The energy may be partially absorbed
    e. All of the above

17. A photoelectron is created when a photon:
    a. Strikes another photon
    b. Knocks an electron out of an atom
    c. Strikes a nucleus
    d. Knocks a proton out of an atom

18. The probability of a photoelectric interaction is higher with:
    a. High-energy x-rays
    b. Low-energy x-rays
    c. Atoms with low atomic numbers

19. Secondary x-rays that result from photoelectric interaction:
    a. Have high energy levels
    b. Cause film fog
    c. Have low energy levels
    d. Occur from photons hitting an atom's nucleus

20. Which of the following interactions is useful in diagnostic imaging?
    a. Photoelectric
    b. Classical scattering
    c. Pair production
    d. Photodisintegration

21. In Compton scattering an x-ray photon:
    a. Loses all its energy
    b. Is diverted by hitting an atom
    c. Becomes an ion
    d. Strikes lower shell electrons

22. As the energy level of the incident x-ray increases, the probability of Compton scattering:
    a. Is zero
    b. Decreases
    c. Increases
    d. Remains unchanged

23. Which of the following is a major cause of film fog?
    a. Secondary x-ray
    b. Compton scattering
    c. Pair production
    d. Photodisintegration

24. What is the effect called when a photon enters an atom and it does not have enough energy to knock out an electron?
    a. Photoelectric interaction
    b. Compton scattering
    c. Pair production
    d. Classical scattering

25. Which of the types of interaction between x-rays and matter have *no* clinical relevance for the imaging process?
    a. Photoelectric interaction
    b. Compton scattering
    c. Classical scattering
    d. Photodisintegration

26. Of the three characteristics of x-rays, which is *not* desirable in producing diagnostic images?
    a. Absorption
    b. Penetration
    c. Scatter

27. If the kVp setting is set too high:
    a. Too much penetration will occur
    b. Too much absorption will occur
    c. Only soft tissue will be visible
    d. The film will be clear

28. Differential absorption refers to:
    a. Limiting penetration
    b. Limiting absorption
    c. Balancing absorption and penetration
    d. The number of rems

29. The measure of the energy of a moving electron or x-ray photon is measured by the unit:
    a. Rad
    b. Rem
    c. Roentgen
    d. Electron volt

30. Changing the kVp setting will change what?
    a. The focus of the image
    b. The kinetic energy of projectile electrons
    c. The degree of filtration
    d. The rads

Answer Key

Answers to Pretest

1. c

2. c

3. b

4. b

5. a

6. c

7. a

8. d

9. b

10. b

Answers to Review

1. Projectile, unstable, higher, photon

2. K, L, binding energy, x-ray photon

3. L, lower, higher

4. Kinetic, reduction, x-ray photon

5. Quantity, quality, intensity

6. Projectile electrons, anode, kVp, increase

7. Quantity, quality, glass window, low-energy, penetrate

8. Photon, inner, photoelectron, binding

9. Electron, absorbed, binding, ion

10. Low-energy, electron, excitation

11. Nucleus, positron, electron, annihilation

12. Matter, high, unstable, proton

Answers to Learning Quiz

1. Gamma rays, the high-energy radiation resulting from nuclear reactions.

2. The level of x-ray energy varies from shell to shell because the binding energy is different for electrons in different shells. The innermost shell, the K shell, has the highest binding energy, followed by the second shell, the L shell, and so on.

3. No, all atoms have different binding energies for different electron shells, and different atoms have different energy levels at different electron shells.

4. There are two reasons why there are fewer high-energy characteristic x-rays. First, only a high-energy projectile electron has enough energy to knock a K-shell electron out of its orbit to produce this characteristic x-ray; not all projectile electrons have the same level of energy. Second, the projectile electron is more likely to miss the electron of the target atom than it is to hit it, since there is much open space inside the atom through which the electron travels.

5. An ion is an atom with a charge because of a missing or extra electron—in this case a positive charge because it lacks one electron. This means that this atom is likely to bond with another atom to create a new molecule. Most such effects inside the body are harmless, but if the altered molecules happen to affect the DNA of a cell, cellular reproduction can be affected in negative ways. Although the photoelectric effect is necessary to produce x-ray images, it is also desirable to minimize excessive ionization within the body.

6. Because high-energy photons result in poor diagnostic images, pair production is avoided in diagnostic radiography since it can be damaging to molecules. Although this is typically not a hazard in radiography, therapeutic radiation used in the treatment of some cancers involves higher levels of energy and may cause pair production interactions.

Answers to Applications

1. The electron from the M shell. The x-ray energy is the difference between the binding energy of the K shell and the shell from which the electron jumped down. In this case a jump from the L shell would be 58.5 keV but from the M shell it would be 66.7 keV.

2. The answer is 2.8 keV, or 69.5 minus 66.7.

3. In this case the photon comes from the loss of kinetic energy. The projectile electron has great kinetic energy as it approaches the nucleus. Since the nucleus has a positive charge and the electron has a negative charge, there is an electrostatic attraction between them. This pulls the electron closer to the nucleus, even though its momentum continues to carry it forward in a bending line. The pull of attraction also slows the electron so that it loses kinetic energy. This energy is emitted as an x-ray photon.

4. If the kVp setting is too high, there will be too much kinetic energy in the projectile electrons. This diminishes the production of the desired characteristic K-shell x-rays.

5. The increased number of electrons will still have the same energy levels, and the quality of the beam will not increase even though the quantity does.

6. Filtration occurs when the x-ray beam passes through the glass window of the x-ray tube or other filters. As it passes through these filters, low level x-rays are eliminated. This process increases the overall energy level of the x-rays.

7. In Compton scattering the atom with which the photon interacted becomes an ion. Ionization is significant in the body because the atom is changed and is likely to bond differently with other atoms, having molecular, and possibly biological, effects.

8. Scattered x-rays can travel in all directions, striking anything in the area in addition to the film. This is one reason radiologic technologists do not stand near the patient undergoing radiographic imaging, because radiation can be scattered away from the patient in all directions. In fact, Compton scattering can occur at any point as the x-rays leave the x-ray tube, being scattered by parts of the equipment such as filters, the housing, the x-ray table, or the floor—anything the x-ray photon strikes.

9. The electron volt (eV), the roentgen (R), the rad (also called gray [Gy]), and the rem (also called the seivert[Sv]).

Notes

Notes

Notes

Notes

Notes

Notes

Notes

Notes